Intermittent Fasting Mastery

Live a Healthy Life by Following This Complete Guide that Many Men and Women Have Followed, for Transforming Their Lives with the Power of Fasting and the Ketogenic Diet!

By Georgia Bolton

Table of Contents

with the express written consent from the Publisher. All additional rights reserved.

The information in the following pages is broadly considered a truthful and accurate account of facts and as such, any inattention, use, or misuse of the information in question by the reader will render any resulting actions solely under their purview. There are no scenarios in which the publisher or the original author of this work can be in any fashion deemed liable for any hardship or damages that may befall them after undertaking information described herein.

Additionally, the information in the following pages is intended only for informational purposes and should thus be thought of as universal. As befitting its nature, it is presented without assurance regarding its prolonged validity or interim quality. Trademarks that are mentioned are done without written consent and can in no way be considered an endorsement from the trademark holder.

Introduction

Congratulations on downloading this book and thank you for doing so. This book will help you in understanding the fascinating concept of intermittent fasting and the health benefits it can bring into your life.

Intermittent fasting is a simple concept of managing fasting and eating hours within a day. However, this simple concept can bring amazing changes in your life. This book will explain all the benefits of following intermittent fasting routine and the ways to do so.

This concept has gained great fame for its ability to help in fat burning and weight loss. But, the health benefits of this method are far beyond the small scope of weight loss. It is a way to gain holistic health.

This book will cover the various intermittent fasting protocols in great detail and would also explain other health benefits of following them.

This is a comprehensive guide on intermittent fasting which will tell you each and every aspect of intermittent fasting that you need to know.

You will not only get to know the ways to follow intermittent fasting for successful weight loss and other health benefits but also tell you the things to avoid.

It will tell you the best eating pattern to have while practicing intermittent fasting, the diet that helps in fat burning most and the foods to eat for best results.

You will get to know the different fasting schedules for men and women and the reasons why they should be different.

From best practices to follow during your fast to the right nutrient mix, everything has been given the due weight in this book for making things clear to you.

The safety of practitioners while following intermittent fasting has been given special attention. You will get to know the precautions to take while following intermittent fasting and the things to avoid during your fasts.

You will also get to know the side-effects and the ways you can know if you are heading in the wrong direction.

You will be able to understand the common misconceptions regarding intermittent fasting and why they do not stand the test of reasoning.

To sum it up, this book is your comprehensive guide to understand the power of intermittent fasting and the ways in which it can bring a positive change in your life.

There are plenty of books on this subject on the market, so thanks again for choosing this one! Every effort was made to ensure it is full of as much useful information as possible. Please enjoy!

Chapter 1: Intermittent Fasting—Plain and Simple

It is easy for successful ideas to become an enigma. People start feeling that if something is working and producing amazing results, there must be a great mystery behind that. It has happened with the concept of Intermittent Fasting.

Intermittent Fasting has emerged as a craze in the past few years. It is one of the most effective ways to manage or bring down weight. It can not only help in reducing weight, but it is also very effective in bringing down the belly fat. This charismatic ability of intermittent fasting is earning it a great fan following.

Intermittent Fasting Isn't a New Discovery

It is important to get this fact out of the way at the outset. Intermittent fasting may have resurfaced in the public domain recently, but it is not a new concept discovered by some weight loss guru recently. The basic concept of intermittent fasting has been the way of life for our ancestors for the better part of humanities existence. Yes, you read it right. It has been the existential way of living for our ancestors for thousands of years.

Our ancestors started as hunter-gatherers where they were always on the move. The food availability was scanty, and hence they regularly faced the periods of feasts and famines. That was a time when neither the food storage facilities were available nor there was any knowledge to do so. Therefore, even if they managed to hunt something big, they couldn't store it for long. The natural process of decay and decomposition rendered the food unusable. They had to start fresh most of the time.

It was also the time when they had little advantage over the animals. It is an established fact that we are neither very fast nor very strong. We can't see in the dark as most animals can. We also don't have long claws or teeth. All these things made us inferior. Therefore, hunting is a skill we perfected over a very long period of time. But, before we got skilled in the art of hunting, the availability of food was largely dependent on chance and weakness of the prey.

All this meant is that our ancestors had to go without food for long periods. Whenever they got food, they had to eat as much as they could in one go. The human body has got adapted to this process, and it works very efficiently in this feast and famine cycle. This is the whole concept of intermittent fasting.

Intermittent fasting means that you will get an eating window in which you can eat a reasonable amount of food. Then, there would be a fasting window in which your body will have to go without food. However, during the fasting window, our body starts to function more efficiently as it is very important for survival.

The modern intermittent fasting concept is a refined way of following that cycle of feasting and fasting for better health and functionality. A lot of health issues including the problem of obesity can be resolved by following intermittent fasting.

Origin of Most of the Modern Health Issues

Most of the health issues faced to a very great extent these days have become very severe in the past few decades. Unhealthy lifestyle and poor eating habits are to be blamed for these problems to a very great extent. We have unknowingly turned the boon of food abundance into a bane and that is the main reason behind most of the problems.

The mid-20th century witnessed a great boost in industrialization. We started producing things on a very large scale. Food security improved considerably at least in the developed world. People had more resources, higher financial resources, and the easy availability of food. Bringing food to the table became easier and we overexploited this luxury. We gave in to the pleasures of food, and this has led to most of the problems that trouble us today. There is no control in the amount of food we eat and the number of times we eat it in a day. The physical activity has gone down, and consumption of calories has increased, and this imbalance has led to most of the health issues.

This is a very simplistic explanation of the issue as several health issues also contribute to the problem, but it is important to understand that unregulated eating pattern is at the base of most of the troubles. In this book, we will be discussing all those issues and the ways in which they can be resolved.

Intermittent fasting can help you in resolving these issues as it addresses the core problems and things start to fall in place on their own. If you are troubled with health problems like obesity, diabetes, high blood pressure, and heart ailments, intermittent fasting is the one-stop solution for treating or managing most of the troubles.

The Things That Make Intermittent Fasting Such an Effective Way to Improve Health

Modern medicine has developed by leaps and bounds in the past century. It has found ways to treat some of the most complex health issues. It is working towards finding the cure for deadliest issues like AIDS, Cancer, Cardiovascular damage, and other such problems. However, it is still unable to find a cure for common health disorders like diabetes, high blood pressure, and obesity. There are ways in which you can manage diabetes, blood pressure, and obesity; however, it still doesn't focus on curing these problems completely. The main reason behind this failure is that modern medicine is always busy in treating and suppressing the symptoms. It seems treating these problems completely isn't very profitable for the healthcare industry in the long run.

The doctors explain excellent strategies to manage problems like diabetes, high blood pressure, and obesity and give medicines to keep them under check. However, they fail to explain the strategies to treat these problems completely. All these issues mainly arise when we make compromises with our eating habits and lifestyle. We are reluctant to change our ways, and these problems keep on getting serious. Medicines can help in keeping the symptoms of these diseases low, but they can't change your lifestyle and eating habits and that's why these problems keep on increasing with time.

Intermittent fasting, on the other hand, helps you in bringing a positive change in your eating habits and lifestyle. This has a very profound effect on the things that cause the problems and hence, treating the issues becomes easier.

This book will cover most of these health issues, and the impact intermittent fasting can have on these problems. It will explain the ways in which you can overcome these problems and have a very healthy and fit body that will be able to fight most of these problems on its own.

What Intermittent Fasting Is and What It Isn't

To begin with, intermittent fasting isn't a diet. It is a lifestyle change that can help you in treating the underlying causes of most of the health issues. It is a very subtle, easy, and effective way to address the functional issues your body is facing. It doesn't require calorie counting, reducing the amount of food you eat or starving yourself. It also doesn't ask you to make time taking preparations or spending large sums in taking meticulous classes. It is a simple way of returning to the roots as far as your eating patterns are concerned. Bringing a change in the way you eat, number times you can eat, and the periods in which you can eat is what constitutes intermittent fasting routine. Most importantly, intermittent fasting is a routine and lifestyle change. If you are ready to make some small change in your eating patterns, most of your health issues can be resolved or brought under control, and the way to do so is intermittent fasting.

The Reason for Ineffectiveness of Other Popular Weight Control Measures

Over the course of the past few decades, diets and calorie restrictive regimes have become quite popular. They boast of their amazing abilities to lower the weight and their impact on other health issues. However, the stats tell otherwise. Most people practicing any kind of diet have experienced that diets become ineffective after some time. They need to go on tougher plans, and it becomes impractical. Around 80% of the people who have been on a diet at one point gained more weight than they had originally lost once they got off the diet plan.

There had been several other measures in practice to lose weight. A significant rise in the obesity graph has also led to growing concern in people about its deadliness. In fact, the Centers for Disease Control and Prevention (CDC) report states that out of 900,000 preventable deaths reported annually in the US have around 400,000 cases which could have been prevented if weight could have been lowered. Obesity isn't simply a cosmetic problem as most people think; it brings with itself a number of problems which can become fatal. So, if one manages the weight properly, chances are that untimely death can be averted to a great extent.

This knowledge has caused great concern about managing obesity effectively and thus have surfaced various ways to control it. From gyms to pills and surgeries, people are ready to try almost everything. However, most of these things have largely proven ineffective in reducing obesity pandemic. Global obesity stats show that in spite of so many weight loss measures in practice, the number of people falling in the obese category has tripled in the past four decades. The weight loss industry, on the other hand, has gained a market value of $68 billion in the US alone in this period. If you include the market worth of the European weight loss industry too, the figures reach around $127 billion.

The reason behind the steep rise in the obesity rates despite so much expenditure lies in the fact that most of the popular weight loss methods are difficult to follow in the long run; they require constant work and devotion of time and money. Something or the other is always missing, and hence people fail in keeping their increasing weight in check.

The thing that makes intermittent fasting so effective is the fact that it is easy to follow. Treats the root cause of the problem. Can be practiced without devoting extra time, money, and attention.

Impact of Intermittent Fasting on Your Weight and Overall Health

One very important thing to understand is that you must not consider intermittent fasting as merely a tool to reduce weight. Weight loss is a by-product of improved health which comes naturally. Intermittent fasting is a holistic way to treat most of the health issues causing trouble in your body. Unhealthy lifestyle and poor eating habits cause havoc in your body. They impair your body function and slowly start to interfere with various crucial functions. These ultimately lead to weight gain and other health issues.

Did you know that you can improve your chances of remaining healthy and physically fit simply by increasing insulin sensitivity in your body? Poor eating habits lead to a serious problem called insulin resistance which ultimately leads to diabetes. The main reason for this problem is frequent eating. It means that if you control the frequency of your meals, you can prevent this major trouble. Once your body falls in the trap of insulin resistance, your weight would start increasing uncontrollably. Any number of weight loss efforts would prove to be ineffective if you develop insulin resistance. It will not only cause diabetes and obesity but will also lead to problems like hypertension, high cholesterol, heart problems, chronic inflammation, and other such issues.

Intermittent fasting is one of the most effective ways to prevent insulin resistance. In fact, it can help in converting the negative state of insulin resistance to positive state of insulin sensitivity. If you have higher insulin sensitivity, your body will automatically work towards fighting weight problems and help you in remaining healthy.

Intermittent fasting is also very helpful in improving your body's ability to fight diseases. It helps your digestive system. It improves your cognitive function and you start gaining more muscles while your body loses fat. It means that you will not only get slimmer but also stronger.

Intermittent Fasting Types—Different Paths to Reach Good Health

One of the best things about intermittent fasting is that it allows you to choose the way you want to follow it. It isn't rigid in practice. If you feel that you want to start slow, you can choose an easy intermittent fasting style that will help you in losing weight. Once you get comfortable with the fasting schedules, you can choose longer fasting routines for better and faster results.

All types of intermittent fasting routines have one thing in common and that's their ability to address the inherent problems that lead to poor health. It doesn't matter if you run on a very tight schedule and can't find time to prepare labor intensive diets or sweat for hours in the gym. Intermittent fasting allows you the flexibility to improve your health and lose weight by simply following healthy fasting and eating schedule. If you find it difficult to resist the temptation to eat a few things, you can still lose weight by following intermittent fasting. It doesn't put severe restrictions on the things you can eat and can't eat.

If you can only fast for 2-3 days in a week and that too only for a few hours, you can follow the easier intermittent fasting schedules. If you want to build muscles, intermittent fasting schedules can help you in reducing the body fat faster and gaining muscles.

It means you can choose a suitable intermittent fasting routine as per your convenience and ability to attain the goal of good health. There are several ways to choose from and every way has its specific advantages.

Types of Intermittent Fasting Routines or Protocols

1. **The Leangains Method—16:8 Intermittent Fasting Protocol**

    This is one of the most popular intermittent fasting protocols, and it gets its name due to its ability to help you gain muscle mass while you keep losing the body fat. It is easy and very sustainable in practice. Your body can easily get adjusted this schedule and follow it on a long-term basis without much trouble.

2. **The Warrior Fasting—20:4 Fasting Protocol**

    As the name suggests, this intermittent fasting protocol is suitable for the big boys and girls. It is one of the most popular fasting routines within the bodybuilding community and people involved in performance sports. It is very effective in enhancing the production of adrenaline and growth hormones in your body that improve your strength and stamina. It also helps in bulking muscles and lowering the fat in the body.

3. **Eat–Stop–Eat Method**

    It is an effective way to lose weight and reduce the risk of several lifestyle disorders without severely changing your lifestyle. If you strongly believe in the advantages of reducing your overall calorie intake but can't follow diets or practice intermittent fasting on a regular basis, this can be one of the best intermittent fasting plans for you. You can fast for any two non-consecutive days of the week and eat in a healthy manner for the rest of the week. The results shown by this method have been very promising.

4. **Alternate Day Fasting—24-Hour Fasting Protocol**

   You can consider this fasting protocol as the regular version of the eat-stop-eat method. It requires fasting for the complete 24 hours and then eating normally for the next 24-hours and then resuming the fasts for another 24-hours. In simple words, you will be fasting every other day. This fasting protocol is definitely for the tough souls, but the rewards are handsome and plenty.

5. **The Fast Diet—5:2 Diet Protocol**

   This is an odd one out when it comes to actual fasting as it doesn't require you to remain in a complete fasted state. This is more of a calorie restricting method for 2 non-consecutive days a week. However, the results of this method have been great, and this has led to the inclusion of this method in the book.

6. **Spontaneous Meal Skipping**

   This is also not a real intermittent fasting protocol, and it isn't structured at all. It is a simple way to listen to your body and skip meals whenever you are not feeling very hungry. However, even skipping meals occasionally can have a very positive impact on your health and that's why this method has got a mention in the book.

We will be discussing all these methods and the correct ways to follow them in detail. You will get to know the specific advantages of each method, and reasons these methods are so effective in their areas.

Chapter 2: Studies that Prove the Effectiveness of Intermittent Fasting

Intermittent fasting may be the oldest way of living humanity has ever known, but scientific research on the subject is very new. The science never paid much attention to the fact that people may be falling sick more due to overeating than malnutrition.

However, this ignorance hasn't been widespread. There are several cultures and religions in the world that have feel following various fasting routines since centuries. They have accepted it as a religious practice to ensure that it is followed by everyone and the whole society can lead a healthy life.

Fasting Followed as Religious Practice and Its Scientific Significance

The reasons for fasting have been different in most religions but it has been invariably present in each one of them.

The Ramadan Fast of the Muslims

Muslims all over the globe observe a mandatory fast for a period of one month every year. In this fast, they begin their fast early in the morning and end the fast after sundown. It gives them 14–16 hours of fasting time while they are leading an active life.

Several studies conducted on the Muslims practicing the fast in these months have proven that their insulin and blood sugar levels improved significantly.

Practitioners lost weight in the months of Ramadan.

Their total cholesterol levels and triglyceride levels also decreased. Women also saw a significant increase in the levels of HDL, the good cholesterol.

The immune system improved in the practitioners, and there was no impact on their kidney function and urine component.

Intermittent Fasting Routines of the Jains

Jainism is a religion practiced in India. It has incorporated intermittent fasting as a way of life for its practitioners.

In this religion, all the followers are expected to eat anything only after saying their morning prayers. This puts their breakfast time around 8-9 in the morning.

The Jain community is a pure vegetarian community, and hence they don't eat anything heavy.

This is a pre-dominantly trader community, and their lifestyle is mostly sedentary. They can eat normally during the day. However, their last meal of the day has to be before sundown. It means most people have their dinner before 5-6 in the evening. They can't eat anything after that.

This gives them 15-16 hours of fasting window.

The rules are the same for men and women; however, the children are not expected to follow this routine.

The advantages:

This is a business community which is involved in very little physical work.

Yet, the community has managed to stay healthy for thousands of years now due to their lifestyle.

They have been following the routine for so long now that it isn't an inconvenience for anyone. It has become a lifestyle.

Study Conducted in 2007 for Prevention of Chronic Diseases Through Alternate Day Fasting

This study showed that intermittent fasting had been effective in lowering the blood pressure in animals.

On animals, it was also noted that alternate day fasting had been effective in reducing the impact of cancer on animals.

However, not much research has been conducted on human beings, and hence the conclusions cannot be drawn.

Studies conducted on some human subject suffering from Type-2 diabetes showed variable results.

A Study Conducted in 2013 to Understand the Impact of Fasting on the Reproductive System

This study was conducted on rats, and it showed that rats when put on fast, demonstrated sexual dysfunction. The impact was more prominent on the female rats.

This is a reason women are advised not to fast for long.

However, this study needs to be done further on human subjects too as the time frame to which the rats were subjected could have been very long when extrapolated in terms of human time as per the respective life cycles.

A Study Conducted in 2017 to Understand the Benefits and Effects of Intermittent Fasting

This study demonstrated that the subjects stopped signs of persistent hunger after a few days. The results of weight loss were, however, inconclusive.

The Intermittent fasting has been a very under-researched subject. Science has now started taking more seriously when promising results have started to come. However, it should never be forgotten that it is an age-old, time-tested way of life and has helped humanity sail through the toughest of times.

Chapter 3: Benefits of Intermittent Fasting

Intermittent fasting is a holistic way to treat your body. Its benefits are no way restricted to weight loss. In fact, as I have stated earlier, weight loss is simply a by-product of the good health that you acquire through intermittent fasting.

Intermittent fasting has a profound effect on several health parameters, and it helps in improving the functioning of your body. Your overall health biomarkers would start improving as soon as you begin your fasting. You would start noticing significant changes in the way your body functions and also in your energy levels.

This chapter will explain the changes in various areas in your health and the reasons for those positive changes.

Improved Insulin Sensitivity

Insulin sensitivity is a term that will be used several times in the book, and therefore, it is important that you clearly understand its significance in your health. Insulin is one of the most important hormones in your body. It has some crucial jobs to perform that affect your weight and fat accumulation too.

Insulin is a hormone released by the pancreas. It performs several functions, but two important jobs performed by it can mean life and death for all of us.

Whenever you eat anything, the food is processed by your body, and it is converted into glucose. The glucose is a ready form of energy that your cells can absorb and use immediately without the requirement of any further processing. So, the process is simple, the glucose mixes in your bloodstream and raises the blood glucose levels. The blood travels all over your body, and hence the glucose is made available to each and every cell of the body to utilizing the energy. The mitochondria in your cells can use this glucose for running the cell functions. However, there is a catch. The cells cannot absorb glucose on their own. There is a barrier that stops them. It's like the cells are locked and they need a key to open them for absorbing the glucose. Insulin is that key which allows the absorption of glucose by cells.

So, the first job of insulin is to bind with the cells and allow them to absorb glucose. Without insulin, your cells will be unable to absorb glucose and starve.

The second crucial job of insulin is to bring down high blood sugar levels. Consumption of food increases the release of glucose into your body. This elevates your blood sugar levels. This is a process that gets repeated after every meal. Insulin lowers the blood sugar levels by storing the excess glucose in a form of glycogen and fat in your body as consistently high blood sugar levels for long can be fatal. It is the main fat storage hormone in your body.

If you fear the accumulation of bulging tires around the abdomen or flapping thighs, then also, this is the hormone you should worry about messing around. This is a hormone which isn't good neither when it is abundant nor when it is in short supply.

It is a very important hormone. You stand no chance of healthy survival if there are any problems related to insulin in your body or the insulin levels are off the chart.

However, I digress. Let us go through the energy process once again. Every meal that you consume ultimately releases glucose. It takes your body anywhere around 8-12 hours to utilize the glucose in the bloodstream and normalize the blood sugar levels. As soon as the blood sugar levels go down, the insulin levels also dissipate. The pancreas in your body will keep producing and pumping insulin as long as the blood sugar levels don't get normal.

Problem #1

It begins with the habit of frequent snacking and having late night meals. The thing is that your cells can't accept glucose on their own. They need insulin to unlock them. It acts as a messenger that helps in glucose absorption. However, when you start having meals every few hours, insulin is always present in the blood. The cells get so used to the insulin that they stop responding to it readily. This is called the incremental threat effect of overexposure. It means that if there is a healthy exposure to a thing, the reaction would be positive, this is called the mere exposure effect. However, when the exposure becomes constant, everything starts developing a distaste. They become insensitive.

This is what happens with the cells. When the insulin is always present in the blood, the cells stop showing their receptiveness to bond with the insulin. This means that although the blood sugar levels in your bloodstream are high, and the insulin is also present, the cells don't show great receptiveness to insulin. Hence, your blood sugar level remains high, and your cells also don't get proper glucose. This is an alarming problem. The pancreas senses the high blood sugar level, and it starts pumping more and more insulin. For utilizing the same amount of blood sugar, your body starts needing much more insulin. This problem is called **Insulin Resistance**.

It puts a lot of pressure on your pancreas and also leads to a problem called prediabetes which is a primary stage of diabetes.

Problem #2

Once you develop insulin resistance, the levels of insulin also remain very high in your blood. Insulin is also a fat storage hormone. It means that by the time the insulin levels are high, your body will not start burning body fat in any condition. You may run on the treadmill for hours, but you wouldn't be burning fat. You would at the most exhaust the glucose in the bloodstream but wouldn't be able to metabolize fat. Therefore, burning fat would remain a big problem in the case of insulin resistance.

Problem #3

There are several hormones that can help in fat burning. However, the production of these hormones can only take place once the insulin levels go down. If your body has insulin resistance and you are having frequent meals, that is not going to happen anytime soon.

Problem #4

Because your cells stop responding to insulin readily, the pancreas has to produce more and more insulin. This puts an unnecessary load on the pancreas. It can also lead to the development of pancreatitis.

Problem #5

Consistently, high blood sugar levels can become a cause of great concern. It can cause fatigue, swelling, and several other serious issues including multiple organ failure.

Insulin resistance is a problem that needs to be feared. There can be several reasons behind insulin resistance; however, frequent snacking is a big one among them.

How Intermittent Fasting Helps in Developing Insulin Sensitivity

The biggest contribution of intermittent fasting to your health is that it helps in the development of insulin sensitivity. The main reason behind the development of insulin resistance is its overexposure to the cells. It happens as your body needs to constantly pump insulin to stabilize the blood sugar levels.

Following an Intermittent Fasting routine would involve remaining in a fasted state for a considerably longer duration. Let us consider the 16-hour fasts as they are one of the easiest routines to follow.

Now suppose, you started your day at 7 in the morning.

Had your breakfast around 9 in the morning.

Had your lunch at 1 in the afternoon.

Finished your dinner by 5 in the evening.

This is the time your fasting window would begin.

You finished your 8-hour eating window. Your body takes anywhere between 8-12 hours to stabilize the blood glucose levels. It means that your insulin levels would start getting low after 5-6 hours of your last meal. Between 8-12 hours, the insulin levels would reduce considerably. However, the fasting window is of 16 hours. This means that your body will maintain low insulin levels anywhere between 6-10 hours. This gives your cells time away from constant insulin badgering at their doors. This is the simple, most important thing that would help your cells in developing insulin sensitivity as the problem of overexposure of insulin would end. The next time when you have your meals, the cells would respond better to insulin stimuli.

Therefore, intermittent fasting can help in a big way in the development of **Insulin Sensitivity**.

Faster Fat Burning

Fat burning is a very unique process. Your body can run on two types of fuel viz. glucose and fat. The food that we eat is mainly composed of carbohydrates, protein, and fat. Your body processes the food that you eat and converts it into glucose. Glucose is an easy to burn fuel, and your body loves to stay on it.

The fat stored in your body isn't toxic waste. Your body has passed through a great deal of evolution to learn to store fat. It can use this fat to provide energy when the ready form of energy from glucose is not available. It is a part of the survival mechanism of your body. However, your body will never start burning fat without a cause. It likes to keep it stored for the times when you are really short on energy. Hibernating animals use their body fat to survive for months while they are sleeping in adverse conditions.

However, to make your body use the fat as a form of energy, you will have to starve it for a considerable amount of time and cut-off the ready supply of energy. This is where intermittent fasting comes into play.

Before we move any further, you will have to understand the mechanism of fat burning.

When you are eating frequently, your body keeps getting the ready supply of glucose. It doesn't matter whether you lower the supply of energy or not. Until your body is getting glucose, it would not burn fat. This is where the diets fail to hit the nail.

People have a misconception that if they lower their calorie intake, their bodies will have no other option than to burn fat for energy. Remember, diets and calorie restrictive regimes only reduce the calorie intake; they never completely cut the supply. When your calorie intake gets low, your body senses that there is a problem. If it keeps running on the normal calorie consumption mode, it will be starved of energy. This is where it makes a move and lowers your metabolic rate. It means that it lowers the amount of energy you require to run your body. This is a reason people start feeling lethargic, tired, and energy drained when they are on diets. However, the body doesn't burn the fat as it simply can't. You lower the amount of food you consume in the meals, but you still have a greater number of meals in a day at short intervals. This keeps your insulin levels high. It is a fat storage hormone, and hence till it is present no fat burning would take place.

Following intermittent fasting helps you in cutting off the energy supply completely at least temporarily. However, your body needs energy supplies at regular intervals as cells can only store small amounts of energy. To run the vital functions, your body has no other alternative than to metabolize the fat stores for providing energy and hence the fat burning takes place.

To initiate fat burning, you will need to stop the continuous supply of energy even in small amounts. This is what intermittent fasting does. It imposes a curfew on ready glucose supply.

When you remain in the fasted state for a bit longer, your body also starts the production of some fat burning hormones. Hormones like the Human Growth Hormone (hGH) and adrenaline are produced that also speed up the fat metabolization. It is important to note here that these hormones cannot be produced by your body till there is insulin present in your bloodstream.

The production of hGH also increases when the levels of "Ghrelin" the hunger hormones are also high. This is also a condition which intermittent fasting fulfills as you remain hungry for long.

Therefore, you can lose weight and burn fat faster by following intermittent fasting protocols.

Impact of Intermittent Fasting on Heart Health

The heart is one of the most vital organs in our body. It pumps blood day in and day out. However, it is a very sensitive organ. Various processes in your body have a very profound impact on the health of your heart. For instance, if your blood pressure remains too high, it will put a lot of pressure on the heart and would cause damage to it. If your blood sugar levels remain consistently high, they will lead to stiffening of muscles and that would also lead to heart injuries. From chronic inflammation in your body to chronic stress, all these things cause injuries to the heart and the vessels carrying blood to the heart.

TV advertisements, product sales scripts, and even medical science have led us to believe that cholesterol deposits in the heart vessels lead to heart issues. Cholesterol blocks the blood carrying vessels and that causes most of the problems. Therefore, you must lower your consumption of fat and cholesterol. The whole concept is misleading, and they are telling only one part of the story.

It is correct that most of the heart problems are caused due to blockage of the heart vessels by cholesterol. However, cholesterol is not the kind of villain it is projected to be. In fact, it is very important for the proper functioning of your body.

Did you know that it is the material from which most of the cells are made?

Did you also know that most of the important hormones are made from cholesterol?

Did you know that cholesterol is the repairing material for your heart?

Whenever your heart vessels get damaged due to high blood pressure, chronic stress or any other kind of injury, cholesterol rushes to repair the damage. It gets deposited on the artery walls as plaque. When the damage is frequent, the plaque deposit gets thicker and leads to heart attacks. However, it was never the primary reason for heart problems in the first place.

Another common misconception is that by removing the fat and cholesterol from your food you can prevent heart damage. It is not entirely true. Dietary cholesterol plays a very insignificant role in causing heart damage. It is simply used for providing energy. Most of the damage is caused by the LDL, VLDL, and triglycerides which are bad cholesterols. Their production is high when the levels of antioxidants go very low in your body, and your body has very high levels of blood sugar.

Intermittent fasting helps your body in improving the overall health biomarkers that lead to heart injuries. It plays an important role in lowering the levels of LDL, VLDL, and triglycerides as they are used by your body to produce energy when the glucose supply is low.

You can give a great boost to your heart health by doing regular exercise as it helps in making the vessels carrying blood to your heart more flexible.

A healthy lifestyle with low stress also helps in reducing the injuries to the heart.

Some of the Important Roles That Intermittent Fasting Plays in Ensuring Improved Heart Health Are:

Promotes Insulin Sensitivity

Insulin resistance is among the leading reasons for common heart injuries and blockage. When your insulin levels remain high very consistently, it directs a lot of harmful lipids to your heart walls that lead to blockage. Insulin resistance also leads to chronic inflammations and that produces cytokines which add to the problem. It is also responsible for high blood pressure which is a major cause of heart damage.

Intermittent fasting is very effective in reversing insulin resistance and that helps in controlling the problems that cause heart damage.

Helps in Controlling High Blood Pressure

High blood pressure is like the cat which is very difficult to tame. It can occur due to a number of reasons. However, one big reason for high blood pressure is insulin resistance. Once your insulin levels are under control, it gets easier for you to manage your blood pressure. The more you have control over your blood pressure, the lower will be the damage to your heart. High blood pressure can also occur due to problems like water retention in the body. Intermittent fasting can also help you in taking care of this issue as well.

Better Stress Resistance

Stress also plays an important role in causing damage to the heart. Intermittent fasting plays a very important role in lowering the risk of damage from stress. When you do any kind of fasting, you expose your body to lower levels of stress. This stress acts as positive stress, and it enables your heart in absorbing stress at low levels. Therefore, when blood pressure, insulin resistance, and other such things cause stress, your heart is better equipped to handle it and doesn't show a shock reaction. Hence, sudden damage due to stress is low.

Reduces the Amount of Free Fatty Acids

Free fatty acids also cause the highest amount of blockage in the arteries. The free fatty acids are released by the visceral fat stored in your body. The higher the amount of visceral fat, the greater would be the amount of free fatty acids. They can cause great damage. However, free fatty acids are not produced without reason. Your body can use them for producing energy under the right circumstances, and intermittent fasting helps in the creation of such circumstances.

Intermittent fasting creates short energy demands in your body. When there is no other source of energy, your body can use these free fatty acids for producing energy, and hence the risk from them will reduce. On the contrary, you will be able to benefit from them.

The Boost in the Production of Human Growth Hormone (hGH)

The Human Growth Hormone (hGH) is one hormone that can make a huge difference in your weight loss efforts. It is a hormone that your body produces to achieve several growth goals.

The production of growth hormone is very high in kids as they are growing. It reaches its peak when they reach teenage as their bodies start growing very fast. However, once a person crosses the teenage, the rate of production of growth hormone gets low as one isn't growing anymore and only aging.

It is a hormone that plays a very crucial role in burning fat, brings anti-aging effects, and healing injuries. These are the reasons that the production of this hormone never stops completely; it simply gets low. Your body produces the growth hormone in short bursts.

The production is very high in the following conditions:

1. When the insulin levels in your blood are very low
2. When you are sleeping and hungry

3. When you do high-intensity exercise

4. When you face any injury or trauma

The fourth condition is not applicable as you wouldn't want to increase your hGH levels at the cost of an injury. However, the other three conditions get fulfilled when you follow intermittent fasting.

Intermittent fasting leads to the development of better insulin sensitivity, and hence your blood glucose levels stabilize faster. This would mean that the insulin levels also start getting low at a better rate. The fasting also ensures that you remain empty stomach for longer, and this also facilitates the production of hGH. In the last legs of your fasting, you are mostly asleep, and hence the hGH production increases. If you couple that with some high-intensity exercise, your body will be able to produce hGH in high quantities.

This hormone can burn fat faster than anything else. It specifically helps in burning fat and building muscles. A study conducted by the American College of Cardiology shows that intermittent fasting can lead to an increase in production of hGH up to 2000% in men and 1400% in women.

Some advantages of high hGH levels are:

- ✓ Faster burning of the abdominal fat tissues
- ✓ Better muscle buildup

- ✓ Increase in stamina during high-intensity interval training
- ✓ Better immune system
- ✓ Better mood regulation
- ✓ Strong anti-aging effects
- ✓ Faster healing of injuries
- ✓ Increase in libido
- ✓ Higher production of anabolic hormones

Therefore, you can burn the belly fat faster if your hGH levels are high.

Better Satiety Through Improved Leptin Sensitivity

Have you ever wondered why people who are obese tend to have a higher appetite? This is beyond reason as these are the people who should eat the least as their energy demands are low. Yet, they find it difficult to resist food when it is in front and that keeps adding on weight to them.

If you have been laughing at them or pitying them, then you are wrong. It is something beyond their control. All this happens when one hormone gets out of control and starts messing with the brain.

The fat cells in the body release a hormone called "Leptin." This is the satiety hormone, and its main job is to instruct the brain to stop eating as the fat stores are high. The higher the fat content in the body, the greater would be the release of leptin hormone, and you should start feeling full faster. However, this is where the problem begins.

When a person has too much fat, the release of leptin is also very high. The problem starts when there is inflammation in the fat cells. This causes the fat cells to keep releasing the leptin hormone at moderate levels all the time. This means that your brain is constantly getting the message to stop eating as the fat stores are abundant. The problem of overexposure starts creating a problem here too. When the release of leptin is constant, your brain stops registering its signal.

The levels of leptin should be the lowest when you are hungry and highest when you are full. The inflammation in the fat cells leads to the moderate release of leptin all the time, and hence brain is unable to distinguish the signal. This is a state called leptin resistance. That is why obese people never feel satisfied. They can eat immediately after eating something.

There are three factors that cause leptin resistance:

1. **Consistent Release of Leptin Hormone:** If your fat cells remain consistently high, your brain would stop registering them, and it would lead to leptin resistance.

2. **Inflammation in the Fat Cells:** If there is inflammation in the fat cells, they would keep releasing leptin, and it would also cause leptin resistance.

3. **High Amount of Free Fatty Acids:** High-fat deposits in the body release more free fatty acids. They can interfere with the ability of the brain to recognize the leptin hormone and that would also lead to leptin resistance.

There are 2 main ways in which Intermittent Fasting helps:

It Stops Chronic Inflammation: Intermittent fasting plays a crucial role in fighting inflammation in your body. It helps in bringing down the free fatty acids which are the main culprits behind inflammation. The lower the inflammation, the greater will be leptin sensitivity. Bringing down free fatty acids also helps in the cause as they stop misleading the brain.

Lowers the Release of Leptin Through Extended Fasting Hours: When you fast for longer hours, your leptin levels go down automatically as the constant release is sparked by frequent eating. When your brain doesn't have to bear the constant knocking of the hormone, it gets better at recognizing it.

The more sensitive your brain is to leptin, the lower will be your urge to eat anything. This will help you in fasting as well as managing weight.

The villain of this story is "Sugar." I started the topic with an unusual thing. The reason is that the ghrelin hormone is supposed to be the good hormone. It performs several crucial functions like makes you feel hungry when your stomach is empty. It also boosts the production of growth hormone. High ghrelin levels can also boost your cognitive function. Your body would be able to regulate insulin better, and your heart would also function better if your ghrelin release is normal. However, that doesn't happen, and the reason is sugar.

The ghrelin is your hunger hormone. When your stomach is empty, the levels of ghrelin are the highest. As you keep eating your ghrelin levels go down, and you stop feeling hungry anymore. The release of ghrelin and leptin is inversely proportional. When the ghrelin levels are high, your leptin levels should be low. When your leptin levels go high, the ghrelin levels must go down as you would start feeling satiety by them. However, that also doesn't happen and that is also due to sugar.

When you feel hungry and your gut starts producing ghrelin you eat. However, if your food of choice is any kind of sugar-laced product, you would be getting empty calories that would raise your blood sugar levels but wouldn't give your gut anything substantial to process, and hence it would keep releasing ghrelin.

The leptin levels remain consistently moderate if you keep eating sweets as they are a reason for inflammation. So, even after eating a lot, your leptin levels would never rise too high. The gut would not get a message to lower the ghrelin levels. You would overeat and load too many empty calories that would also cause obesity.

Consistently, high levels of ghrelin would slowly start decreasing the impact of the hormone and all other functions would get affected.

Intermittent fasting helps you in putting a stop although temporary to consistent loading of sugar into your system. The longer you remain away from sugar, the better your ghrelin release would be. Remember, this hormone affects the functioning of several other hormones and functions and messing with it can be dangerous.

Reduction in Chronic Inflammation

Chronic inflammation is dangerous. It can lead to problems like heart diseases, hypertension, thyroid issues, obesity, chronic pain, diabetes, migraines, and even cancers. Not only this, problems like autoimmune diseases like ulcerative colitis, rheumatoid arthritis, multiple sclerosis, and Crohn's disease are also caused by chronic inflammation.

High amounts of oxidative stress, free fatty acids, triglycerides, LDL, and VLDL in your blood lead to chronic inflammation.

The risk of chronic inflammation increases if:

- You are overweight
- You eat unhealthy things
- You are leading a stressful life
- You have a sedentary lifestyle

Intermittent fasting can help you in managing the oxidating stress and free fatty acids. It also helps your body in using up triglycerides, LDL, and VLDL in your blood for producing energy. This lowers the risk of chronic inflammations, and you can avoid these problems.

Intermittent fasting is a healthy way of living, and it also helps in reducing your weight which in itself is a reason for inflammations. Better lifestyle also lowers the risk.

Help in Diabetes

In general, all the diseases are bad. They limit your capabilities and take the fun out of life. You lose time, money, and health. However, those diseases are especially bad for which there is no permanent cure.

They simply stick to you. They become lifelong disorders, and diabetes is one among such problems.

Serious and poor management of diabetes can have serious implications. We all know that high blood sugar levels are bad, and they can even cause multiple organ failures and death. But low blood sugar is not any less dangerous. It can cause seizures, coma, or even death. Therefore, proper management of diabetes is crucial.

The problem with diabetes is that it simply sticks with the patients for the whole life. It means that the patient becomes dependent on medications and insulin injections. Conventional medicine has no other way to treat this problem.

Intermittent fasting can be a savior for people suffering from diabetes or prediabetes. The US alone has more than 110 million people with diabetes or prediabetes.

It isn't without fact that intermittent fasting can help in lowering the impact of diabetes or reversing it. To make it clearer, it is important to understand the underlying causes of diabetes and the ways intermittent fasting helps in them.

Helps in Maintaining Healthy Blood Sugar Levels

High blood sugar is the main problem in diabetes. Your body cannot bear high levels of blood sugar. It causes microhemorrhage in the eyes, kidney, and heart vessels. This means that the vessels in these organs start to leak blood. To counter that, a special type of protein material called fibrinogen increases in your blood that leads to clotting. However, excessive clotting of blood can cause obstructions in the vessels carrying blood to heart, kidney, and eyes. Strokes, high blood pressure, impaired vision, and hardening of the arteries are some of the immediate effects. It ultimately leads to organ failure if blood sugar levels do not come down. High blood sugar also leads to fatty liver and may also cause liver cirrhosis.

Intermittent fasting helps in this area a lot as it reduces the risk of frequent blood sugar spikes. Your blood sugar rises every time you eat food. It is the result of glucose from the food mixing in your bloodstream. Intermittent fasting limits your eating windows, and this lowers the risk of frequent blood sugar spikes. Additionally, following a high-fat low-carb diet is also important. It helps your body in running on fat fuel rather than glucose provided by carbohydrates.

Helps in Decreasing Insulin Resistance

Insulin is the main hormone that regulates your blood sugar and puts it to good use. As soon as your blood sugar increases, the pancreas starts off-loading insulin to help in the absorption of that blood sugar. The real problem begins when the cells stop responding to insulin. This is a problem that can happen due to overexposure of insulin, and it is called insulin resistance. In that case, the pancreas needs to pump more and more insulin even for absorbing small amounts of blood sugar. Additional insulin shots may also be required to fulfill the need for insulin. The solution to this problem is that your body needs to become more sensitive to insulin. However, our eating habits act against developing insulin sensitivity. People wrongly believe that if they stop eating sugar, their blood sugar levels would go down. This is not going to happen. Either you eat sugar or not, if you are eating, your body will convert it into sugar, and your pancreas will keep pumping insulin to process it.

This is where intermittent fasting can come to the rescue. It helps in bringing prolonged fasting hours where food intake completely stops. Your blood sugar levels go down in 8-12 hours and so do your insulin needs. Around 16 hours of fasting creates a gap of 4-

8 hours when your bloodstream was free of excess insulin. It helps in the redeveloping of insulin sensitivity. Your body starts responding better to the insulin produced by the pancreas and doesn't need extra insulin to be injected.

Gives a Chance to the Pancreas to Recover

Excessive production of insulin puts the pancreas under a lot of stress. The pancreas has very important functions. It produces insulin, glucagon, and various enzymes. Extra burden on pancreas can lead to several complications. Pancreatic insufficiency is one among them. This will lower the ability of the pancreas to produce insulin, glucagon, and enzymes.

Intermittent fasting helps by giving your pancreas the time to recover. The time when you are not eating during intermittent fasting, your pancreas does not need to pump more insulin. After a certain amount of time, your body needs to burn fat and for that, the pancreas produces glucagon. This changes the function. Created insulin sensitivity and pancreas can also recover.

Helps in Weight Loss

It is an open secret that weight loss is among the most effective ways to successfully manage diabetes. Intermittent fasting leads to weight loss in a number of ways and, therefore, gives you much-needed respite from the harmful effects of diabetes.

Promotes Anti-aging

We all want to stay young forever. We know that's an unreasonable demand, but something simply snatches away our youth much earlier than it should go, and I believe there is nothing more unreasonable than that. People consider early aging only to be a cosmetic issue, but it isn't. Aging is much more of a physiological problem too. Aging occurs when the damage to your body is higher than the normal rate at which it can regenerate things. The regeneration process slows down as we grow, but it has accelerated at an early age then you are looking for the problem at wrong places.

Three most important reasons for faster aging are:

- High free radical damage
- Oxidative stress
- Low Glycosaminoglycans (GAG) levels

You already know that intermittent fasting can help you in reducing the free radical damage and oxidative stress. The GAG is a chemical that is responsible for keeping the collagen of your skin hydrated. Once the levels of GAG go down, your skin starts to wrinkle and sag. This GAG production is controlled by another hormone produced in your liver by the name of IGF-1. Intermittent fasting is the only known way to boost the production of this hormone.

Autophagy

Autophagy is a new term that has come in the limelight as a Japanese scientist by the name of Yoshinori Oshumi recently published his research on this matter in 2016 and won a Nobel prize for it. This concept states that your body has an innate ability to treat most of its problems on its own. The only thing required is the right conditioning.

Our lifestyle these days has become such that we are providing everything to our body in excess. This has made our bodies inefficient in its functioning as it doesn't need rationing. However, our body has the ability to run more efficiently if it is forced to do so.

He states that in case our body senses a shortage of supply of energy, the first thing it does is that it starts optimizing all the processes. It is important for running the body longer on less energy. This process of optimization of the processes is called autophagy.

The beauty of this process lies in the fact that it doesn't waste anything and starts using every part of your cell to regenerate new cells. It even starts purging all the pathogens, germs, harmful bacteria, and fungi in your body as they are also using up energy. Most of the problems start getting resolved in the process.

It means even the toughest physiological problems and chronic inflammations will get treated on their own if your body starts the process of autophagy.

The requirement for autophagy is that you must temporarily cut the energy supply of your body from outside. It means you must stop eating. When you eat, you are not only feeding your body, you are also feeding all the pathogens, infections, chronic inflammations, cancer cells, and other malice.

Intermittent fasting can help you in starting the process of autophagy. It gives your body the required break it needs and that's why intermittent fasting is so effective in treating most of the problems.

Some people believe that actual autophagy only starts when you fast for long. However, studies have shown that autophagy can also begin when you fast for shorter durations like 12–16 hours.

This process can take you toward good health and intermittent fasting can be the way to achieve it.

Chapter 4: Intermittent Fasting Protocols

As we had discussed earlier, intermittent fasting is simply a pattern of fasting and feasting. The health benefits would largely depend upon the number of hours you fast, the kind of food you eat, and the lifestyle you follow.

Intermittent fasting in itself is a complete method. It means that if weight loss is a goal, you will achieve it irrespective of the fact that you exercise, or you don't. You will lose belly fat even if you are not able to ditch the fast food completely. However, these are the factors which have a significant impact on your weight loss speed. Therefore, if you are following a healthy lifestyle, doing a bit of exercise and eating healthy, your weight loss journey would be a lot smoother and faster. You will also be able to remain healthy and fit for longer with very little extra effort.

Weight loss is a very small part of the advantages that intermittent fasting has to offer. We have discussed all the health benefits that you can get by following intermittent fasting routines, and hence you must keep them in account while comparing intermittent fasting with any other diet plan.

You can keep shorter and easier fasts or go for tougher fasting protocols; the choice would always be yours. However, you must always remember that while you can tax your body, you must not try to challenge it. Our bodies don't like getting shaken to a jolt. The reactions are sometimes intense. From steep hormonal changes to erratic reactions, your body may react in abnormal ways if you will try to take up something to which your body isn't accustomed. Therefore, you must always start with easier intermittent fasting schedules and then move on to the next one when the body gets used to it.

The Preparation—Getting Rid of the Habit of Snacking

If there is one thing that has caused the highest amount of damage to our health in modern times, it is the habit of frequent snacking. Some so-called came up with the idea that frequent snacking habits keep the metabolism running, and the food producing industry started pushing it with its full might as it suited their business. The more frequent the snacking habit is, the better their business would be. It helps the cereal making companies, it helps the companies that produce ready-to-eat products, and it even helps the fast food industry.

The benefits of frequent snacking were pushed so hard through commercials and campaigns that people started treating it as gospel truth. Probably the saying "A lie told often enough becomes a truth" is true after all. However, it is one of the main reasons behind the obesity epidemic plaguing the whole world today.

The habit of frequent snacking is also one of the biggest roadblocks you will face that deters people from fasting or staying hungry. We are actually habitual of a dangerous cocktail. First, we like to eat frequently at very short intervals. Second, most of the times, the essential component of these snacks is refined sugar. These two things lead to cravings for food. It means you will keep on feeling the need to eat even after short food intervals. These needs are called food cravings and initially, they make remaining in the fasted state very tough.

So, to follow intermittent fasting in a proper way, you will have to try to ditch these two things as much as possible. If you can completely leave them well and good, or else, try to maintain a safe distance and don't let them overpower you.

The best way to prepare your body for intermittent fasting is to eliminate the snacks from your schedule completely. It means that you will have to manage with only 3 meals a day and nothing besides that. It looks tough and let us examine the reasons that make it tough.

On any given day, we all have got into a habit of eating 6–8 times a day. For some people, the number of times they eat in a day can be even higher. However, if we consider the number of times that we spike our insulin levels in a day, the instances can go as high as 10-15 times. Before you let this settle in your mind, you must also remember that every time your insulin levels are spiked, your fat burning abilities diminish considerably. Your body becomes more eager to accumulate fat than to burn it. The insulin spike in your body would take place every time you ingest anything that contains calories. It means sipping a cup of tea, coffee, or soda can spike your insulin levels. Not only this, chewing a sweet gum, a candy, popcorn, or anything else containing calories will also have the same effect. Now, considering all these facts, put some pressure on your brain and try to recollect the number of times you caused insulin spike yesterday. If you have reached a higher number than we have discussed, I won't be surprised.

On average, our eating schedules go as follows:

No.	Description	Time
1	Pre-Breakfast snacks	6-8 am
2	Breakfast	8-10 am
3	Morning Snack	10-11 am
4	Lunch	1-2 pm
5	Evening Snack	4-5 pm
6	Dinner	7-10 pm

| 7 | Post-Dinner snacks | 9-11 pm |

These are the times when we are eating things that are loaded with calories. Our meals are full of refined sugar in various forms that also aggravates the problem. Higher the number of times you eat in a day, the more difficult it will get for you to remain in the fasted state.

The first thing that you must do in order to follow any kind of fasting schedule in any considerable manner is to eliminate all kinds of snacks from your food. There is no getting around this point. If you have a habit of frequent having frequent snacks, you will experience powerful cravings that will be difficult to avoid. You must eliminate the snacks from your routine and stick to 3 meals a day routine. This will help you in fighting with cravings, and your system will be able to get better at treating insulin. If you are not able to stay away from snacks, fasting may get very difficult for you to follow, and food will always remain the main thing at the back of your mind.

The Leangains Method—16:8 Intermittent Fasting Protocol

This is one of the most famous intermittent fasting protocols. As I have already told, this intermittent fasting protocol gets the name Leangains from its ability to help you in losing fat and gaining lean muscle mass. Both of these things have been unheard of in the weight loss industry till now. The methods which caused any amount of fat loss also undoubtedly led to the loss of muscle mass too. The reasons for the same are simple. When you start restricting energy supply to your body, the first thing it tries to use for energy is the most similar looking structure, and protein definitely fits the bill. Carbohydrate is the easiest to break and a favorite fuel of your body. After it, comes protein, and the fat is always the last choice as your body requires a completely different process to burn it.

The Leangains method compels your body to start burning the fat. The fat in your body is a very stable fuel. Burning even a small amount of fat can provide a lot of energy, and it releases the least amount of toxic waste. However, your body can't keep burning carbohydrate and fat at the same time. So, while your body is really burning the fat, there will be no substantial loss of the muscle mass. In fact, if you engage in high-intensity interval training while practicing intermittent fasting, you will be able to build muscles faster as it helps in the production of two important hormones called the growth hormones and the adrenaline. Both these hormones greatly enhance the ability of your body to build muscle and stamina. So effectively, your body would lose the fat accumulated at your belly and thighs and build muscles.

After you have been practicing intermittent fasting for a while, you might notice that you weigh almost the same on the scale although you are feeling you are getting slimmer. If that is the case, there is all the reason for you to be happy as your body would have adapted itself to the fat burning process. It would be burning fat and that would make you get slimmer. However, you also start to gain muscle mass. The muscles are more compact and heavier than fat and that's why although you may look slim you may not weigh less but it is a blessing in disguise and the dream of millions.

The Process

This method is called the 16:8 fasting protocol, and the reason for it is that you will need to remain in the fasted state for 16 hours a day and have an eating window of 8 hours. This schedule is for men who want to follow this protocol. For women, the ideal protocol would be 14:10 with 14-hours of fasting window and 10-hours of eating window. Several studies conducted on women have shown that shorter fasts work better with the hormonal system of the body of a female. So, although this protocol is popularly known as 16:8, it is effectively 14:10 for women and that shouldn't be confused.

The Fasting Window

This is the time people are worried about the most. Although 16 hours of fasting may look like a big number, by managing your eating schedule well, you can pass it very easily.

The most important things about easily passing the fasting window are the timings of beginning the fast. It is always the best to time your fasts as per your morning routines. If you like to wake up early in the morning, then you must try to begin your fasting early in the evening. For instance, if you wake up at 6 in the morning, then your fasting must begin by 6–7 in the evening at the latest. The earlier it begins, the least amount of restraint you will have to apply on your urge to eat something.

The 16:8 Fasting for Morning People

Suppose you begin your fasting at 6 in the evening. If you are a morning person and wake up early, you will have to sleep early. This means you will go to bed by 10–11 at night. This would give you 4–5 hours of gap between dinner and sleeping. This is an undisputed fact that having dinner a few hours before going to bed is the best for your health. Having dinner 4–5 hours before the bedtime makes it highly probable that you will remain in a physically active state. It will also make the digestion process faster and smoother. By the time you will go to bed, food processing in your body would be nearing its completion stage, and it is among one of the best things for your body.

The 4-5 hours before you go to sleep would be easy as you'd feel no real urge to eat during this time. Starting the fasting at 6 would mean that by 7 in the morning you would have passed a majority of the time effortlessly in your sleep. Women would only need to continue their fasting for another hour and for men, there would be 3 more hours to pass before they can break that fast.

Once you start practicing intermittent fasting, you would stop feeling the urge to eat anything specifically in this time as your body gets used to the routine and your gut starts timing the release of 'ghrelin', the hunger hormone, as per your eating schedules. However, if you still feel the hunger pangs, you can have unsweetened black tea, black coffee, green tea, or fresh lime drink without sugar. These beverages would help you in suppressing your hunger without adding calories to your system. These are not only safe beverages but also provide a lot of antioxidants. You must try to continue your fast for as long as possible as the longer you would continue your fasting, the better would be the results.

The last few hours of fasting are crucial for fat burning. This is the time when the production of the hGH and adrenaline is at its peak in your body. These two hormones can help you in burning fat big time. Even a small amount of exercise will lead to terrific results.

I'd highly recommend exercise during this period. If you can do high-intensity interval training, it is the best as it leads to faster fat burning and muscle buildup. However, if you don't have the time or inclination to do that, even simple cardio exercises, aerobics, or yoga would also be very beneficial.

The women can break their fast after 14 hours, and men can do that after 16 hours of fasting.

Your eating window should ideally begin after the given hours of fasting. However, there is no reason to be very rigid about the timing. You can take the liberty of an hour if you feel the hunger to be uncontrollable and try to fast for longer the next day. This is something that would feel tough initially but would become effortless later on.

The Eating Window

The eating window should be of 8 hours. However, you must try to limit the number of times you eat in these 8 hours. Intermittent fasting is all about managing the number of meals and hours, it doesn't lay very great emphasis on the things you eat. It is natural to expect anyone trying to lose weight to eat healthy things. So, you should avoid eating fast food and food items rich in refined sugar. Most processed items or so-called low-fat food products are high on sugar. You should try to avoid them. But, you don't need to count calories if you are eating healthy things.

The Breakfast

This should be the heaviest meal of the day. You will be entering the most active phase of the day and would also be ending your fasting schedule. Therefore, it is very natural for you to feel very hungry. You can treat yourself with a good meal. However, the best tip for your breakfast meal would be to have a high-fat and low-carb diet. The fat gives more energy but is very slow to burn. This means that by having a high-fat diet, you will be able to go without food till your lunch effortlessly. You wouldn't feel the urge to have snacks in between and that is our goal.

The meals high in carb get digested very fast. They provide instant energy but would make you feel hungry very soon. It is best to avoid such items that are very high in carbs. The protein should be the second most important part of your meal after fat. You should consume moderate amounts of protein. It also takes longer to get processed, and it is very important for building muscles. However, you must avoid overdoing protein as that would do no good to you. If your diet is too high on protein, it would also start adding too many calories.

Therefore, 65-75% of the calories from your meals should come from fat, around 20% of the calories should come from protein, and only 5-10% of the calories should come from carbs.

The carbs that eat should only be things that are rich in fiber. It means you should only try to eat whole grain foods, non-starchy green leafy vegetables and things like that which have very high digestive fiber content.

The Lunch

It is the second meal of the day, and you should try to keep it very healthy. Eating fiber-rich food items like salads and fruits is always the best as it keeps you feeling light and fresh. A very heavy lunch often makes people feel drowsy.

The Dinner

This should be the lightest and healthiest meal of the day. People have a misconception that if they don't eat much in the dinner, they won't be able to make it through the fasting window easily. This has no basis. In fact, if you have a very heavy dinner, you are most likely to face problems like indigestion and food cravings.

This meals should be rich in digestive fiber. The digestive fiber takes very long to get processed while it adds very few calories to your system. This would mean that you will not feel hungry for very long after having your dinner.

If you are a morning person, never try to start your fasting late at night.

The more you delay the time of the fast, the longer you would have to remain in the fasted state in the morning. That is mostly very difficult for people.

The 16:8 Fasting for the Late Nighters

If you are a person who likes to burn the midnight oil, then beginning your fasting early in the evening wouldn't be such a great idea for you. However, this shouldn't mean that you can have it around midnight. Always try to time the beginning of your fasting window 4-5 hours prior to your bed-time. Going to bed immediately after having dinner can be very bad for your health.

You can have your dinner around 9 pm so that you can have your first meal of the day at noon. Everything else remains the same.

Intermittent fasting doesn't impose any hard and fast rule on you. The way you want to manage your food and lifestyle would always be up to you. However, it is expected of you to follow strict eating and fasting windows as they help in the regulation of your insulin levels, hGH, ghrelin, leptin, and several other hormonal levels. The timing is also very important for ensuring the good health of your digestive system and other vital organs.

The 16:8 intermittent fasting is the easiest to follow as it can be turned into a schedule. Your body adapts to its routine very quickly and times the feasting and fasting patterns. It is a very easy and sustainable way to live your life. You can make it a part of your life and may never feel the need to change it. It doesn't require you to make any other significant change in your lifestyle other than changing the hours you remain in the fasted state. It is simply like shifting your breakfast time a bit farther.

It is the best intermittent fasting schedule for all those people who have been repenting their inability to pay any special attention to their health. All those people who regretted their inability to take time out for exercise, diets, and meal planning can follow this routine and have all the health advantages with minimum effort. The 8 hours of eating window gives you complete freedom to eat literally anything as long as you are showing responsible behavior and reasonable restraint.

So, if you had been cursing your increasing weight, abdominal fat, and inability to do anything about it, this fasting routine gives you the chance you had been waiting for.

The Warrior Fasting– 20:4 Fasting Protocol

As the name suggests, this fasting schedule is for the people who have the warrior spirit. First, let us understand the significance of its name.

Our ancestors lived the lives of warriors. In fact, for every meal, a war was fought. Their food was the biggest foe. The animals they preyed upon were faster, stronger, and more capable than them. Getting food was uncertain, and most people traveled far to get their prey.

This meant that the probability of getting food was generally once in a day. The Braves went in search of food and when they returned with the prize, the whole group could have food only after that. This led to natural longer fasting. However, eating only once a day didn't make them weak. On the contrary, science has proven that your mind becomes more focused when your body has been running without food for around 24 hours. The physical instincts also get sharper. You are able to respond better and react faster. These were the abilities that helped them to hunt the animals which were better equipped than them. Fasting for longer increases the adrenaline rush in your body, and your stamina increases. You are able to endure fatigue better and test the physical limits of your body.

The same lifestyle is the inspiration for the 20:4 intermittent fasting schedule. The warrior fasting is the most popular schedule for bodybuilders and people involved in performance sports. It helps them in increasing their stamina and strength. They can do their workouts for longer and have a good supply of natural hGH and adrenaline in their blood. This is the reason they are able to achieve such extreme levels of low body fat and high muscle mass. They train for hours at end and don't face severe exhaustion.

The Process

The warrior fasting requires you to continue your fasting state for 20 hours at a stretch. Although it may look like that 4 hours is enough to fit two meals, but they aren't. It is very unlikely to have a second meal within such a short gap especially when you have consumed a very heavy meal with a lot of fat, protein, and very little carb. So effectively, 20:4 fasts mean one meal a day. You can have an elaborate single meal over a broad course which should start with lighter things like soup and then have the real food after a while once your body starts feeling a bit nourished.

Ending a long fast with a very heavy or solid meal is never advisable as it doesn't give your body the time to adjust. Always get off the fast with something light and then get on to heavier stuff. Therefore, the 4 hours given in this schedule are purely for having a simple big meal distributed over a considerably long period.

You can start your fasting whenever you want as there is no way to pass the whole fasting window in the dormant state. However, it best to time most of your workout schedule at the end of the fasting window as the production of hGH and adrenaline would be at its peak by the end. It will help in faster bulking of muscles. You would be able to work out harder and better.

The eating window is also very important as your energy demands would increase significantly, and you would have a considerably short span to consume all the required calories. Your warrior diet must consist of high-fat and high protein diet with very low or no carbohydrates. All the carbohydrates that you consume must only come from non-starchy green leafy vegetable and salads as they only supply fiber and very few calories. High-fat food would help you in going strong for the next 20-22 hours without food as they can provide energy for long. Fat takes a very long time to get processed and keeps you feeling satiated.

Switching to a high-fat diet and long fasting also starts the fat burning process in your body. It means your body starts using your own body fat for producing energy if you have high-fat content. This is a great intermittent fasting routine for all those people who can fit the bill.

However, you should never begin your tryst with intermittent fasting from this as then your chances of failure would increase considerably. This is a pro-routine which requires a great deal of practice and discipline. This routine is very hard to turn into a sustainable habit. It has to be followed strictly as a bulking routine. The warrior routine has several other health advantages too apart from fat loss and muscle buildup.

- It is a very helpful routine for stabilizing your blood sugar levels.
- You will feel more energetic and active.
- It is especially very helpful in improving your cognitive function.
- Warrior fasting is also very helpful in reducing chronic inflammations

It should only be carried out in weekly cycles.

Eat-Stop-Eat Method

This intermittent fasting method involves remaining in a complete fasting state continuously for 24 hours at least twice in a week on non-consecutive days. It means you can fast for a full 24 hours and then eat normally the next day. On the eating days must apply great restraint and not eat unhealthy things or not eat excessively. Then you can fast on any other day in the week in the same manner.

This is a simple and easy to understand intermittent fasting schedule. There are no extra rules. You only need to fast for 24 hours on two separate days of your choice in any given week. During your fasting days, you can have black tea, coffee, green tea, and fresh lime as long as they are unsweetened. As long as you are not adding sugar to these things, they will not break your fast and provide a lot of antioxidants.

These longer fasts have a very positive impact on your health. Besides all other specific advantages that come with intermittent fasting, these fasts also help by initiating the amazing process of "Autophagy."

Although this routine gives you great flexibility to fast on the days of your choice and does not impose the restriction of fasting every day, it is difficult to follow as a routine. Due to the longer duration of the fasts and the long gap in the fasting days, it becomes almost impossible to make them a normal habit for your body. You are most likely to feel the hunger pangs on the days of the fast. Following this routine on a regular basis makes it a bit easy but that doesn't change the fact that your body would go through the churning. However, the stress exerted by this routine is very positive and gives great results.

Alternate Day Fasting—24-Hour Fasting Protocol

Alternate day fasting is also similar to eat-stop-eat intermittent fasting routine in most respects, the only difference being that it is more regular in nature. It means that you will have to follow the fasting and eating days every other day. It means that there will be fasting days when you will have to remain without food for the complete duration of 24 hours. You can eat normally for the next 24 hours in which you will maintain a healthy diet. The next 24 hours will again be observed as the fasting hours, again followed by a day of feasting normally.

This can definitely be a very taxing routine as you will have to observe fasting every other day. However, a good thing about this routine is that it is considerably easy to make it a routine. Although your body would never take 24-hour fasts to be a norm, yet the hunger pangs subside after a period of time, and you are better able to remain in the fasted state.

This routine has amazing health advantages, and it starts running the process of autophagy at a much better speed. You can get visible anti-aging effects and feel much younger in appearance as well as the energy levels.

However, you must remember that this fasting method is not for beginners. Fasting every other day for someone who is not used to fasting schedules is neither easy not suitable. You must first practice the easier routine and only try this once your body has got used to the fasting stress.

The Fast Diet—5:2 Diet Protocol

This is an interesting inclusion in the list as it is not a fasting protocol in the real terms. It is more of a calorie restrictive regime, but it has shown great promise and results and that has inspired me to include this in the list.

It is one of the easiest ways to lose weight and has been very effective for women as it prevents any kind of hormonal imbalance that may occur due to fasting for longer hours.

This protocol involves eating normally within the specified calorie range for 5 days of the week and following a calorie restricted diet on two non-consecutive days of the week when the calorie consumption needs to be brought very low.

For men, the permissible calorie intake on the fasting days should be 600 calories. However, there is no restriction on the number of meals in which you can consume these calories. You only need to ensure that you do not cross this calorie threshold. If you can reasonably divide 600 calories into 3 meals, then this method doesn't object to it.

For women, the permissible calorie limit is 500 in a day. It means that through the course of the whole day, women can consume 500 calories at the most.

This method has been very effective in controlling weight and improving several health biomarkers.

Spontaneous Meal Skipping

This is also not a form of intermittent fasting but a way to increase the gap between your meals so that you can get the benefits of intermittent fasting without having to put up with the routine.

This method says that you must skip your meals whenever you are not feeling really hungry. It is an obvious thing to do if you look at it reasonably. However, you will be surprised if you reconsider your own eating patterns. We all have become so habitual of routines that we do most of the things out of the force of habit. It means when the clock strikes 1-2 in the afternoon and it is officially declared as the lunchtime, you have your lunch. Most of the times, it isn't the hunger that forces you to have lunch but simply a habit.

We also indulge ourselves in impulsive eating when we see others having something or have a food stall in front of us. Those are the times when we aren't hungry at all but still grab a bite. These are extra calories going into your system that can never be used. They are bound to get stored as fat.

Spontaneous meal skipping inspires you to only have a meal when you are actually feeling hungry. If you are not feeling a strong urge to eat, you must skip the meal and not cave in under the pressure of time or habit.

This meal skipping will help your body in developing insulin sensitivity and improve overall health biomarkers.

Chapter 5: Things That Can Help in Making Your Intermittent Fasting More Effective

There are several things that can help your weight loss efforts and health gain efforts while you are following intermittent fasts.

Four important things that can especially boost your efforts are:

1. Balanced Food
2. Good Exercise
3. Adequate Sleep
4. Healthy Routine

We will be discussing the impact of good exercise and the ones to follow in a later chapter, and hence we will be skipping that part in this chapter. It will suffice here to mention that exercise can boost the health benefits of intermittent fasting several times.

Balanced Food

Food is an important part of our lives. We become what we eat. If you look closely, 90% of your physique is simply a result of the things you eat and the manner in which you eat it. This means that even if you are not pumping iron for hours in a gym, you can have a considerably good physique if you are eating balanced food.

The concept of balanced food has been misunderstood to a very great extent. Healthy and balanced food which will have all the required macronutrients. It should have the required amounts of micronutrients, vitamins, and minerals too.

The 3 Macronutrients for Your Good Health

Fat

Fat has been the most essential part of our diet since the very beginning. Our ancestors had no idea of farming. They could only hunt and gather. The things they killed to eat had a good amount of fat and protein. These two things are our basic requirements, and we got them through the meat. This is a reason we survived without difficulty. Even today, most carnivorous animals survive only on fat and protein.

The fat has several crucial functions to perform. It can provide you with long-lasting energy as it is slow burning fuel. Even small amounts of fat can give you energy for long. It packs a punch when it comes to the number of calories in a specific amount of food. Fat has almost double the calories as compared to carbs in weight.

You can eat more fat at a time and store more energy while you will eat the same amount of carbs and get less energy. Fat also provides insulation against cold. It was also a reason our ancestors needed fat so much as fur coats and other clothing material was not at their disposal.

It is a macronutrient that must be a part of your weight loss diet.

There is a general misconception created by the food producing industry that eating fat would make you fat. There is nothing more absurd than this theory. Whatever you eat gets converted into energy in one or the other form. Therefore, fat making you fat and carbs not doing the same has no basis. However, the phobia from fat led to low-fat foods. People are crazy about low-fat foods and that has caused more obesity than anything else.

When fat is taken out of anything, not only the fat goes away but also the things that make the food tasty. Low-fat foods will not have any taste. The food industry can't sell tasteless food and therefore, it adds a lot of refined sugar in various forms to compensate for the loss of taste, and this increases the problem several times. Sugar adds more empty calories, causes cravings, leads to inflammations in the liver and spikes your insulin levels.

Your food must be rich in fat. In fact, 65-75% of the calories you consume in a day must come from fat. High-fat food would ensure that you are able to withstand long intervals between your meals easily. It also helps in beginning the process of ketosis.

Ketosis is the process of burning the ketones in your body. When your body is devoid of glucose energy, it has no other option than to burn the fat.

Your body is equipped to run on both kinds of fuel i.e. glucose and fat. However, it can't run on both at the same time. Now, glucose derived from the carbs is an easy to burn fat and therefore your body prefers to burn it. But it can run on fat if it is devoid a high carb diet.

When you are consuming a high-fat diet with moderate levels of protein and very low levels of carbs, your body starts burning fat for energy and this process is called ketosis.

It is one of the best diets for a person trying to lose weight and fat. This kind of diet is called the Ketogenic diet or the Keto diet. We will be discussing it in detail ahead.

Protein

Protein is important for your body as you need it for building muscles. Every day you lose some muscles and build new ones. For building new muscles, you will need to eat protein as it is the building block of muscles. However, you should only eat protein in moderate quantities as excessive protein would also be converted to blood sugar which you would want to avoid.

The ideal percentage of protein in your diet should be 15-20%. It means of all the calories that you get, only 15-20% calories should come from protein. Lean meats, egg whites, fish, cereals, kidney beans, and several nuts are great sources of protein.

Carbohydrate

Carbs are the primary source of energy we are consuming these days. Most of the weight gain issues faced these days are due to high consumption of carbs. However, projecting all types of carbs as the villain is not correct.

If you are consuming refined carbs then you are definitely going to invite trouble as these carbs get digested very fast and give an instant boost of energy. However, they cannot provide you with energy in the long term or keep you feeling satisfied. Therefore, eating such carbs would lead to food cravings. Sugar laced products also do the same. They add empty calories to your system and cause a great insulin spike. Your body gets a sudden energy kick but nothing for your gut to process. This can act very bad on your digestive process.

However, there are good carbs too. The carbs that you get from whole grains like barley, maze, and other such whole grains contain several important trace minerals that are essential for your body. You need these minerals, and these carbs are a great source. Then whole grain crabs also add a lot of digestive fiber to your system. This fiber plays a very important role in the health of your digestive system.

The fiber helps in cleaning the digestive system as it cannot be digested. It keeps your gut busy for very long, and hence you keep feeling satisfied even with small amounts of meals.

You also get a lot of soluble fiber, vitamins, minerals, and antioxidants from non-starchy green leafy vegetables. You can eat them as much as you want without being conscious about the calorie measurements. They are very healthy, and the soluble fiber forms a gel-like substance in your gut which helps in treating most of the digestive tract issues. The vitamins, minerals, & antioxidants in these vegetables also help you in staying healthy.

If you want to lose weight, the portion of carbohydrates in your diet should be very small. This is not including the non-starchy green leafy vegetables as you can consume them as much as you want. You should limit the intake of carbs from other things and only consume carbs in the form of whole grains and vegetables.

The calorie contribution of carbs should not be more than 5-10% and all of it must come from whole grains and vegetables.

Good Exercise

Exercise is important as it helps you in burning the fat faster. Exercise helps you in creating an extra energy demand. However, as your body is in the fasting state during your exercise, it cannot fulfill that energy demand by burning glucose. This forces your body to burn fat for producing energy and fat burning takes place. This process is very simple, but it cannot take place if your body has a ready supply of glucose. In that case, you will only be burning that glucose energy without disturbing your fat stores ever.

Therefore, it is important that you do all your exercises and especially the high-intensity interval training exercises at the end of your intermittent fasting schedules. This is the time when your fat burning abilities are at their peak.

Adequate Sleep

Giving your body the required amount of rest and sleep is also very important as it helps in proper recovery from the light positive stress caused by fasting and exercise. It is very important that you never ignore this aspect.

Sleep has some very crucial roles to play in your health.

1. The production of the hGH is at its peak while you are sleeping, and it helps in fat burning
2. Your body can produce high amounts of adrenaline in your sleep that will boost your performance
3. Your body carries out a lot of repair and rejuvenation work while you sleep. If your sleep is not adequate, these activities can get affected
4. Lack of sleep can make your body release stress hormones like cortisol. These hormones can stop any kind of fat burning as they push your body in the same mode. If you want to lose weight and remain healthy, proper sleep is a must for you.

Healthy Routine

Following a healthy routine is very important for the smooth functioning of your body. Intermittent fasting is a routine, and the word "routine" is very important here. It is not something that you can one day or one week and you will be able to reap the benefits for your whole life.

Your body goes through changes every day. It faces the challenges every day and therefore, it needs to be treated well on a regular basis. If you are following the intermittent fasting schedule on an irregular basis, you will not be able to stay healthy and fit.

The reason for the great success of intermittent fasting also lies in this very fact that it is a very sustainable way of living life. You can integrate the intermittent fasting in your life and may never need to change anything in your schedule. Therefore, if you want to lead a healthy life, you must make intermittent fasting a routine.

It is also important to have a healthy and active lifestyle. Our weight depends on the simple calculation of the number of calories consumed minus the number of calories burned. If you are living a sedentary lifestyle, you will not be burning any more extra calories than the ones burned by your metabolic processes and fat accumulation would get faster.

Stress is also a big reason for most of the health concerns. The higher the stress you take, the more you are likely to engage in emotional eating and other such activities that also lead to weight gain. If you are facing high-stress or any other kind of emotional turbulence in your life, you must try to deal with it immediately.

Chapter 6: Intermittent Fasting and Keto

Advantages of Keto on Intermittent Fasting

Intermittent fasting and keto diet are a match made in heaven. Both initiate the same process and work towards bringing the same results. The Keto diet involves increasing the fat in your food to the highest levels with moderate proteins and no or very low carbs.

This helps your body in running on fat fuel as the supply of glucose fuel is blocked completely. So, either you are consuming food or burning your body fat, the process remains the same, and the body doesn't have to make the switch frequently. This one thing makes both the processes so compatible.

When you begin your intermittent fasting, you force your body to burn the body fat by cutting off glucose supply. However, if you are on a normal diet, your body would again switch back to burning glucose provided by the carbs. It doesn't happen in case of a keto diet as through food also you get only fat.

Your body starts the effective process called the ketosis. When your body is not getting energy from any other source, the fat cells start releasing the ketones. These ketones can be converted into energy. This process of burning the ketones is called ketosis.

At the beginning of intermittent fasting, people can face several side effects as your body goes through sugar withdrawal symptoms. These symptoms can be a feeling of light-headedness, nausea, and weakness. Although these symptoms are temporary, some people get really worried. Combining intermittent fasting with a ketogenic diet can help you in suppressing some of these symptoms too.

Another big advantage of ketosis is fat oxidation. When your body is constantly burning glucose fuel, it releases a lot of by-products known as AGEs that promote chronic inflammation and oxidative stress.

The tumors in the body are also affected if you are on a keto diet. Actually, the scientists have recently found that the only difference between the functioning of tumor cells of your body and the normal cells is that they cannot survive on energy provided by the fat-rich diet. They lack the components that can metabolize fat. This means if you are on a keto diet, you can literally starve the cells causing and spreading cancer and tumors in your body. All the other normal cells in our body can metabolize fat and therefore, they won't get affected.

You would feel less hungry while on a keto diet. The fat can keep you feeling satisfied for much longer.

Some of the Best Foods to eat while on a Keto Diet:

1. Seafood
2. Non-starchy green leafy vegetables
3. Cheese
4. Avocados
5. Meat and Poultry
6. Eggs
7. Coconut Oil
8. Olive Oil
9. Cottage Cheese and Yogurt
10. Nuts and Seeds
11. Berries
12. Butter
13. Shirataki Noodles
14. Olives
15. Black tea and coffee
16. Dark Chocolate

There might be some symptoms that will show that your body has begun the process of ketosis.

Main Signs Telling Your Ketosis Has Begun

Bad Breath

The level of ketones increases in your blood when your body starts ketosis. This can give your breath a fruity smell. It should indicate that your diet is working for you.

High Ketones in Your Blood Work

Although you will not get to know this change without a blood test if you are following a keto diet and want to know if you have entered ketosis, you can take a blood test. High levels of ketones in your blood will be a testimony to the fact that ketosis has started.

Low Appetite

Once your body enters ketosis, you will notice suppression in your appetite. Your urge to eat will go away. There is no reason to worry about this. It happens because your body starts using a long-lasting fuel. Its need to consume food for short term energy ends. Even if you are not eating anything, the body manages to run its energy supply by burning your body fat and that's why you feel less hungry.

Better Focus and Energy

Fat is a clean fuel and provides cleaner energy without leaving less toxic waste. There is low oxidative stress, and other problem items like the VLDLs and triglycerides are also getting used along with free fatty acids. This leads to cleaner energy. Your brain also starts using this energy and works better. This leads to better focus and high energy.

Fatigue in the Initial Stages

This is a side-effect most people face in the initial stages and worry about. However, there is nothing to worry about. It happens when your body is adjusting to the change in the fuel burning mechanism. If you are feeling the fatigue too much, you should try taking electrolytes. They help in suppressing the symptoms. You should also take sodium, potassium, and magnesium supplements in your daily diet.

Diarrhea and Constipation

These are the real problems that some people face and there is no getting around these problems. Your digestive system has to make a lot of changes when you shift from carbs rich diet to a keto diet. This may lead to these issues. However, these symptoms are also temporary and go away very soon.

Sleep Issues

Sleep issues can become a problem in the initial stages of starting a keto diet. Although this problem is temporary, some people can get restless as they are unable to sleep properly. However, there is no reason to worry as your body would soon adjust, and you will have much better sleep that earlier.

Fat and Weight Loss

There is no doubt in the fact that fat and weight loss is among the most notable symptoms of entering ketosis. The impact of ketosis is visible in your appearance. You would rapidly lose weight and would start to measure less around your waist circumference. This is one sign that you would love.

Chapter 7: Exercise and Intermittent Fasting

Exercise is a sure-shot way to increase the benefits of intermittent fasting. It helps in faster fat burning and also promotes muscle buildup. You can improve your stamina by doing regular exercise and improve your body's response against stress, especially of your heart.

When you do high-intensity interval training, a nitric oxide dump takes place which can catalyze and promote health. It soothes your muscles and helps them in relaxing. This can be crucial for organs like a heart which are generally under high stress.

When you are at the end of your fasting cycle, the production of hGH and adrenaline is at its peak. This hormone can enhance your abilities to do exercise.

Exercise also helps in improving the way in which muscles repair themselves. You can have a faster rate of recovery from injuries if you exercise regularly.

Exercise is also very important if you want to burn your fat faster. It increases the energy demands of your body. Hence, the body has no other option than to burn fat to produce that required energy. This leads to faster fat burning.

Although exercise is one of the best ways to speed up the results of intermittent fasting, some important rules need to be followed. For instance, if you are following longer fasts, then you should avoid doing high-intensity interval training (HIIT) on the days of your fasts. This is due to the reason that your body is in an energy deficit mode, and you may start feeling tired pretty soon.

You must also avoid doing HIIT on consecutive days. This is to prevent overstressing your body. HIIT puts a lot of strain on your body and especially the muscles for which you have done exercise. Doing the same exercises on consecutive days will put an extra burden on those muscles. A lot of muscles break and regenerate after exercise. Continuous stress can cause injuries. There must be days of rest between your exercise days. It will give your muscles the time to recover.

HIIT

High-intensity Interval Training (HIIT) is one of the best ways to make your body burn fat. You can get faster results by investing little time in HIIT. You may have to walk for much longer to get the same results which you can get from small sprints. It also helps in the better buildup of muscles.

On alternate days, do easy cardio exercises. You cannot do HIIT every day. However, on the days you are not doing HIIT, you must do light cardio exercises, yoga, brisk walking, etc. as these activities help you in staying fit. They are good for your heart health and also provide great relief.

You can do weight training on all days if you like as your body wouldn't need to put in much energy effort into that.

Give Your Body Time to Re-energize

This is very important. If you put a lot of stress on your body, it can have adverse effects on your health. Always start slow when you begin your intermittent fasting and then build your stamina as you move ahead.

Walk a Lot

People generally undermine the health benefits of brisk walks as they believe it doesn't lead to weight loss or fat burning. This is a misconception that needs to be broken. In fact, walking has several health benefits:

NEAT Also Uses Up Energy: When you walk or move around even for some time, your body consumes energy. It is like informal consumption of energy coming in short bursts. People do not count it as substantial, but it is. You can burn a lot of energy in this way and it will lead to weight loss.

Helps You in Suppressing Hunger: If you are feeling hungry or your mind is racing towards the thoughts of food, you must go for a short walk. It can help in suppressing hunger for good.

Good for Heart: Brisk walks are very good for the heart. They help in supplying oxygen in good amounts to the vital organs.

Chapter 8: Supplements

Intermittent fasting is a comprehensive solution for most of the health issues. However, when you start following any kind of routine that changes your eating patterns or the amount of food you eat, your body can get deficient in some nutrients. Nutrient supplements can help you in compensating for these deficiencies.

Drink Plenty of Fluids

While you are following intermittent fasting, your body will be a lot of detoxification. It means it will start cleansing itself. It will dump a lot of fluid, and with fluids, a lot of minerals are also lost. This is the biggest loss that happens, and you need to be careful about it.

The first thing that you must do is drink a lot of fluids. However, you should avoid drinking plain water or any kind of soda. The lost fluid had a lot of minerals, and when you drink a lot of plain water, the mineral levels in your body goes down. To prevent any kind of dehydration, you must always mix a pinch of sea salt to your water and it can help you.

Electrolytes

You can also drink electrolytes as they also help in preventing dehydration. You will not feel weak or dehydrated if you are consuming a lot of electrolytes.

Lime

Another way to prevent problems and keep yourself well hydrated is to have unsweetened fresh lime water with a pinch of sea salt. While doing intermittent fasting, it is important that you consume at least one fresh lime a day. You can use it for preparing fresh lime and that would also do the trick. This simple thing can prevent the formation of stones. Actually, when you start fasting, your body starts washing out calcium and other mineral deposits. Some of these minerals can accumulate as stones. Having a lime a day helps you in clearing out these substances from your body.

Potassium

Potassium is also an important mineral that you would need to take. You can get this mineral through natural sources like banana which has a lot of potassium. Pomegranate also has a lot of potassium, or you can also take potassium supplements.

It is important to keep your potassium levels up as it is an important mineral needed by your body. While you are doing intermittent fasting, your body is going through a lot of changes. It changes its fuel source and the way it was functioning. Potassium deficiency can increase problems.

Antioxidants

Chronic inflammations are one of the biggest villains when it comes to poor health. They keep weighing you down and you don't even get to know about them until it is very late. Intermittent fasting plays an important role in preventing chronic inflammations. You can also help in this cause by consuming food items that are high in antioxidants.

Healthy fats, nuts, seafood, vegetables, whole spices, turmeric, and garlic are some of the things which are high in antioxidants. You can take the antioxidants to speed up the healing process of your body. Antioxidants also play a very important role in preventing chronic inflammations.

B Vitamins

B vitamins are necessary, and you can't have enough of them. Taking these vitamins helps in promoting overall health.

Probiotic Foods

Your gut plays a very important role in promoting your health. However, it remains neglected most of the time, and we only pay any attention to it when there are problems related to our gut. Our gut has trillions of helpful bacteria that facilitate digestion of food and healthy digestive tract. However, overeating, acidity, gastric issues, bad foods, and antibiotics are some of the things that can cause great damage to these bacteria. You can help in repopulation of these bacteria by consuming probiotic food.

Magnesium

It is a mineral that our body needs for performing several crucial functions. It is a cofactor for hundreds of enzymes. We can get it from the vegetable green, but most people are usually deficient in magnesium as they don't consume vegetable greens. Its deficiency can affect your blood pressure, heart rhythm, muscle tone, vitamin D absorption, and stress. You can increase your intake of vegetable green for improving the magnesium levels or you can also take supplements to fulfill the deficiency.

Chapter 9: Intermittent Fasting for Women

Intermittent fasting is a great way to reduce weight and that's why it is always a reason for inquiry for women. Women are usually more conscious about their weight and looks than men. They want to lose weight faster and that's why the highest percentage of subscribers to fitness programs are women.

Intermittent fasting has also caught their attention and that's a reason most women start following intermittent fasting without proper research.

Following Intermittent Fasting Like Men Can Be Dangerous for Women

There is no other way to emphasize this fact more clearly. Yes, it is right. If women start following intermittent fasting like men, they can get into a lot of trouble. The reason lies in their own body. Women have a very sensitive hormonal system that can become overreactive if women start remaining hungry for very long without taking proper precaution.

Can't Women Practice Intermittent Fasting?

Of course, they can practice intermittent fasting, and it can have a great impact on their weight. The only thing is that they need to take more precautions than usual. If they start keeping fasts without following precautions, their hormones get off the chart and start giving trouble. They are very sensitive to food. Women may hate to accept it, but the food is not only their physiological need but it also offers emotional and psychological assurances.

The Reasons for the Difference

The reason women need to follow intermittent fasting differently lies in the fact that they have different physiology. Nature has given them the gift of bringing another life into this world in the form of babies. This gift also requires them to be prepared for bearing a child at all times. Their bodies are more sensitive to fat accumulation, and they also have a sensitive hormonal system that reacts adversely to hunger. It means various hormones in the body of a women can go off the charts if a woman starts staying hungry for long all of a sudden.

Nature has made women in such a way that their bodies function better at a higher level of fat in the body as compared to men. Men should ideally have

10-15% of body fat, and they can function optimally at these levels. However, women need around 18-20% of body fat.

Their hormonal system is also very different. A woman's body bears a child. Most of the process of formation of a child takes place with the help of fat. This makes their bodies a bit protective of fat. Besides that, women can start feeling cranky, irritated, hyper, depressed, angry, and many other such things if they go hungry for long. This is also due to the way in which their hunger hormone ghrelin reacts with other hormones in their body.

This makes it necessary that women do not start any kind of drastic fast, calorie restrictive regimen, or diet without proper preparation and precautions.

Precautions for Women Who Want to Follow Intermittent Fasting

- Women who want to follow intermittent fasting must keep some important things in mind:
- Never begin fasting with any strict or longer fast
- Always give their body the time to adjust to the fasting schedules
- They shouldn't test the limits of endurance of their bodies as far as remaining hungry is concerned

- They should take supplements as loss of minerals can have a prominent impact on their health

Things to Remember

- If you want to follow intermittent fasting, always start with the simplest fast.
- Start by skipping the snacks first and then start increasing the time between meals.
- First, you must ensure that all your meals end within 12 hours window and start by practicing 12 hours fast.
- Once your body gets used to 12-hour fasts, you can start the 14:10 fasts.
- Always remain on a specific fasting routine for at least a fortnight before moving on to the next one.
- The 14:10 fasting schedule works best for women. It is neither too long nor short and gives great results.
- Women can also follow the 5:2 fasting protocol as it has also shown to benefit women a lot.
- Women should never keep a fast longer than 24 hours in any condition.
- While men are said to have benefited greatly from longer fasts, they have had adverse results on women.

When to Stop

It is very important that women must know when to stop intermittent fasting. Despite taking all the precautions, a woman's body may not react favorably to intermittent fasting. It can happen due to various reasons, and the biggest one is the different needs of every woman's body. A woman can react completely in a unique manner due to different stimuli. So, if you notice anything abnormal, then you must stop intermittent fasting and consult a physician immediately.

Given below are some of the conditions in which women should immediately stop intermittent fasting.

If Trying to Conceive

If you are trying to have a child, then you must immediately stop intermittent fasting or following any kind of calorie restrictive regimen. Several studies have shown that fasting or depriving the body of food and nutrients for long can cause fertility organs to shrink temporarily. Therefore, if you are trying to conceive, it may take much longer to get successful or you may not be able to conceive at all as long as you are on fasts.

On Getting Pregnant

If you have gotten pregnant, you must stop intermittent fasting immediately. A pregnant woman has very high energy needs. She is making a baby out of the body fat and also needs to nurture the baby with the energy she gets from the food she consumes. Therefore, she should stop intermittent fasting immediately.

While Nursing

If you are nursing a child, you shouldn't follow intermittent fasting for that duration as it may lead to nutrient deficiency. Your body needs more energy and for that, you need to eat properly.

If the Periods Become Erratic

Some women may have erratic menstrual periods due to calorie deprivation. If anything like that happens, you may need to adjust your fasting periods. If the problem persists, you must consult a physician immediately.

If There Are Sudden Changes in Eating Patterns

The eating patterns of some women can get affected adversely due to longer fasting periods. They may stop feeling hungry or may keep feeling famished. If the problems are minor, they must make an adjustment in their eating patterns. However, if the problem is serious a physician must be consulted immediately.

Other Signs Indicating That You Should Stop Intermittent Fasting

- On continuously feeling cold
- When facing acute digestion issues for long
- When you start feeling weak in the heart or have feelings of palpitation
- When the mood swings become very frantic and erratic
- If your skin has started to appear very dry all of sudden or you have developed acne
- If you start noticing sudden and significant hair fall for no apparent reason
- When you start having sleep issues
- When you become very averse to romance all of a sudden
- When your ability to bear the stress of any kind reduces significantly

Chapter 10: The Best Ways to Handle Hunger Pangs and Cravings

Hunger pangs and cravings can be tough to handle at times. When hunger pangs and cravings start taking control of your mind, the only thing that comes to mind is food. Your mind remains fixated, and the time starts to stretch for you. Passing even minutes seems like an hour. You remain seated at one place with your mind wandering around food. This is the times when your digestive system also starts its churning. You start getting a grumpy and growling stomach. To make matters worse, there can be an acute stomach ache. Headache and irritation can also come following all these symptoms. All this could happen because you are having a strong urge to eat. These are extreme scenarios, but they happen with everyone once a while.

However, if you start practicing intermittent fasting you will have to become a pro at handling hunger pangs and cravings for good as ignoring them can make you a regular victim of these problems.

Keep Yourself Busy

It is a very important thing that if you are sitting idle in the fasting period, you will feel stronger hunger pangs, and your mind would wander around food more frequently. The best way to deal with this problem is to keep yourself busy. The more occupied your mind remains, the less it would think about food. Remember that most of the times when you are feeling the urge to eat anything, it is an excuse of your mind to create a diversion from current events or to avoid any work. So, hunger pangs can be easily avoided or tolerated if you are occupied with some work.

Keep Drinking Water

This one is also very important. Water is such a beautiful beverage. You can drink plenty of it and have no consequences. It will fill up your stomach without adding any calories. If you drink enough, you can make hunger go away easily. However, you must remember one important thing, do not drink too much water without adding a pinch of sea salt. Drinking too much plain water can lead to excessive urination, and it would drain you of minerals. So, either drink electrolytes, fresh life water without sugar or add a pinch of sea salt to your water and you can drink it safely.

Eat Fiber and Protein Rich Food

One of the best ways to help you feel satisfied without having unnecessary food cravings is to have a lot of fiber and good amounts of protein in your diet. Protein is heavy and takes time to get digested; this makes it sit in your stomach. Your stomach doesn't feel empty very fast, and you can go without feeling hungry for much longer. Eating fiber-rich food is also an easy and good way to avoid cravings for food. The fiber doesn't get digested and keeps your stomach busy for very long. Therefore, if you fear the cravings of food, then start eating food that is rich in protein and fiber.

Drink Unsweetened Black Tea and Coffee or Green Tea

Black tea, coffee, and green tea are some of the beverages that do not add any calories to your system and hence can be consumed safely during your fasting window. Apart from that, these beverages are rich in antioxidants and help you in fighting several problems. When you begin intermittent fasting, leave sugar, or start a keto diet, you can face symptoms like lightheadedness, weakness, nausea, headache, and other similar issues. These are temporary signs of sugar withdrawal. These beverages also help you in fighting these symptoms successfully.

Don't Remain Awake Until Late at Night

Sleep is very important when it comes to taking the full advantage of intermittent fasting. It helps in fighting various chronic issues, and your body is also able to fight stress and other problems. However, one more thing in which your sleep helps you is fighting hunger pangs. When you remain awake for too long, your brain starts playing with you and gives a feeling that you are hungry. It happens very often, and the best way to fight this feeling is to never stay awake till very late at night. In this way, you will not only be saving your body from overtaxing itself but also escape the hunger pangs.

Use Vanilla Scented Candles to Keep Cravings Away

If your cravings for sweet are very high and you keep feeling like eating sweets, the best way to fight that urge is to light vanilla scented candles in your room. These sweet-smelling candles reduce your cravings for sweets. It works in the fashion of incremental threat effect theory where overexposure to something leads to less likeliness of that thing.

Exercise

Exercise can also help you in distracting your mind from eating. Several hormones are released during exercise that helps you stay away from food. You feel more energized, and your mind also gets distracted.

Go for a Walk

This is also one of the best options to stay away from food. Walking gives your mind a healthy distraction from the thoughts of food. You get a chance to think about other things. It can help you in fighting the hunger pangs.

It is important to remember that hunger pangs are very short. Your stomach releases a hormone called ghrelin when it feels that there is a need for food. This hormone sends the signals to the brain and the brain directs you to have food. However, if you ignore this signal for some time, the ghrelin release would subside, and you would stop feeling hungry anymore. You may have personally witnessed this several times when you had been feeling hungry some time ago, but because it took time to get food, you stopped feeling hungry anymore. So, if you are feeling the hunger pangs and yet it isn't the time to eat, sit tight for a bit and the feeling would subside on its own.

Chapter 11: Ways to Stay Motivated

Weight loss may be a daunting task for which you may be prepared to go to any length. However, staying hungry is also not an easy task either. Most of the people are troubled by their weight when they are in public. Apart from those who have severe health issues, overweight people do not have much of an issue with their weight in close quarters. However, it is not the same as staying hungry. Either you are in public or all alone, staying hungry can make you anxious if you haven't conditioned your mind well. In some circumstances, you may even feel bothered when you are with others.

Pushing yourself to stay hungry and on track isn't an easy task. It is very easy to feel the urge to cheat once a while. However, once you give yourself the leeway, it is very difficult to get back and you see all your effort getting flushed down the drain which can be very sad and demotivating.

This is a battle easiest to fight when there is someone with whom you can share your ordeals or who can provide moral support and the required distraction when needed. If you have a support group, you can ask for advice, share your problems or just even discuss things related to your progress. There can be several ways to have this moral support in your life.

- You can share your journey with your close and understanding friends
- You can discuss your desires with your family
- With other people facing the same problems. You can work as an anchor for each other
- You can also join support groups
- Join online communities

Are Support Groups Really Important?

It depends upon your outlook, the kind of person you are, and the amount of weight you want to lose. If your weight loss targets are normal and you are not facing obesity in real terms, you may do fine even without support groups. If you live in a close-knit family, you may not need to find your moral support elsewhere. If you have close friends who care for you, then you would already have a support group.

However, if you are living alone or facing problems in sharing your concerns, thoughts, and worries, then the support groups may do more good to you than you can think. The support groups can not only provide sympathy and support but they also provide valuable advice, insights, and counseling. There can be several types of support groups to join.

Some Common Types of Support Groups Other Than Your Friends and Family

Commercial Programs

There can be several institutions running weight loss programs and counseling programs. They have their own set of experts who can suggest you better ways to follow your weight loss journey. There are experts to guide you on every step of the way, and hence the journey becomes easier. You have people to look up to and the ones with whom you can discuss the perils in the way.

The success rate of people in these groups is generally high as they find it easy to remain motivated. The experts in the group keep motivating these people and show them the way to move forward.

Enrolling in Clinic-Based Programs

This is a more professional approach to weight loss and other health issues. There are experts to monitor your progress and they keep guiding you on every step. It is always easy to get a professional answer to your queries, and the dangers of things going horribly wrong anywhere are very less as the people handling the progress are actually medical professionals. It is a bit expensive way, but it works, and it is especially very good for you if you are already facing any serious health risk like diabetes, heart problems, or other such issues. Supervision of a medical professional helps you in remaining confident that if anything starts going wrong, an expert is there to guide you.

Volunteer Programs

These programs are run by volunteers and hence they are generally free. Most such programs are conducted for obtaining results for some studies over control groups. These programs offer advice for free, but they monitor the subjects very closely and expect them to follow the set conditions rigorously. In case the subjects fail to meet the desired goals, they can be taken off the programs. Although sticking to these groups might look difficult, their success rates are very high as every subject get individual attention and monitoring. The changes are made from time to time to get the desired results.

It doesn't matter whether you enroll in any kind of professional support group or confide your journey in your friends and family, the important thing is to stick to the protocols and keep making the adjustments.

There will be times when you may find the going getting tough. However, it will still be important to keep going.

Remember, obesity isn't simply a cosmetic problem; it opens Pandora's box of problems. Choosing to live with obesity is choosing to live a life of limitations. You will limit your mental, physical, and emotional abilities. You will make a compromise to live an insufficient life.

Getting obese can occur with anyone, but only those people will remain so who don't show the courage to fight with the problem. Obesity isn't an irreversible handicap, but it does make you less of a person if you stop fighting it.

It will bring a number of diseases which will limit your freedom to do things in life. You may choose to live with diabetes, but you will need to remember that you could have tried to avert it. The same goes for high blood pressure, heart diseases, chronic inflammations, and other lifestyle disorders.

Therefore, it is the best option to stand up for yourself and fight against the malice called obesity.

Healthy living is your right, and nothing can take it away from you if you are determined. Intermittent fasting is one of the easiest ways to fight this big enemy. The only thing required from you is to stay strong in the journey and face the enemy with full might.

Chapter 12: The Good, the Bad, and the Ugly of Intermittent Fasting

Every coin has two faces, and even intermittent fasting isn't an exception. Like every other method, there are some things that can trouble people practicing intermittent fasting. This chapter will explain the good, the bad, and the ugly of intermittent fasting. It will explain the symptoms that will go away very soon. It will also explain the problems which if persist, you may need to make changes. And finally, it will explain the things in the light of which, you must not follow intermittent fasting as that can be risky.

The Good

The good thing is that most of these troubles are temporary. Your body needs to go through some major changes, and the side effects that you may face will be a part of that change and hence, you will stop experiencing those symptoms very soon and hence, if you face them, there should be no reason to worry. You may find these issues to be difficult, but they are minor troubles and wouldn't affect you much in the long-run.

Cravings

Having strong cravings to eat sweets is a common problem people face in the initial stages of intermittent fasting. It would happen more if you continue eating sweets and sugar. These cravings can make you restless, but there is no need to panic as these symptoms will pass away very soon. Eating sweets lead to the release of certain chemicals that make you feel good. However, this feeling is short-lived, and as soon as it passes away, you want to eat more to feel that state of goodness. It is a vicious cycle and leads to no good. Eating sweets will continue adding empty calories to your system that would cause more harm. Therefore, even if you feel the cravings to eat sweet, you must avoid it, and soon, you will find that you don't want to eat sweets anymore.

Hunger Pangs

We have already discussed that hunger pangs are temporary, and the ways to deal with hunger pangs have also been discussed in the chapter earlier. Hunger pangs are temporary, and soon, your body will get used to staying in the fasted state for the set period easily.

Feeling Low

This is a problem that people feel initially. However, there is no reason to worry as this happens when your body is still learning to burn fat for energy. Our bodies have got used to glucose fuel, and they want to run it that way. It is a short-lived fuel and that's why you start feeling low soon after you have consumed your meal. Once your body gets adjusted to ketosis, you will stop feeling low on energy. On the contrary, you will feel more energetic and livelier.

Headache

Headaches are a part of the sugar withdrawal symptoms that would end very soon. You can take unsweetened black tea or coffee once or twice when you feel the headaches and soon after a few days of practicing intermittent fasting the headaches would go away.

Irritation

There can be a feeling of irritation for unknown reasons. It happens due to hunger and sugar cravings. However, the irritation would also not last very long, and you can try to divert your mind to other things to get over the temporary feelings of irritation.

Constipation or Diarrhea

When you start practicing intermittent fasting and keto diet, the food and eating pattern changes drastically. Eating at regular intervals and eating junk have become a part of our lives. However, when you change your diet, your gut takes some time to adjust to the changes. Constipation, diarrhea, bloating, and heartburn are temporary issues. In fact, after a few days of practicing intermittent fasting, you would notice that problems like acidity, constipation, and heartburn would vanish completely. You would be able to process the food very easily.

Feeling Cold

You may at times feel the pores of your fingers and toes to be getting very cold. There is no reason for you to be concerned from this as the problem occurs due to lack of ready energy. The glucose fuel travels easily, whereas it takes time for your body to start moving the fat from your adipose tissues to your pores. However, if your pores have started feeling cold, then it means that your body has started the process, and it will soon start working very efficiently.

Overeating

This is a problem most people face in the initial stages. When they get off the fasting window, they feel famished and eat a lot which may also cause discomfort. This is an adjustment you'll learn to make soon. You will have to follow a bit of restraint when you get off your fast. Overeating can leave you feeling bloated. There is no reason to overeat as your body is already producing energy from fat. To prevent eating more, you must eat slowly. The more time you'll take to eat a meal, the less you will be able to eat as your satiety hormone 'leptin' would send signals to your brain to stop eating. It takes some time for your brain to recognize that you are full, and therefore, if you are eating fast, the chances of overeating increase. Take your time to eat meals, and this problem can be prevented.

Frequent Trips to the Bathroom

You may need to go to the bathroom several times when you start intermittent fasting. This happens because the body starts the detoxification process in the initial stages. You must keep yourself hydrated and drink a lot of water with sea salt and fresh lime. You can also drink electrolytes to prevent the loss of minerals.

The Bad

Fluctuation in Sugar Levels

The blood sugar level fluctuations can be bad. If you are suffering from diabetes, you must consult your doctor in the loop so that your insulin dosage can be adjusted accordingly. In the initial stages, this can happen more. However, there is no permanent solution to this problem. Intermittent fasting is one of the best ways to bring insulin sensitivity, but a problem that has been building for long would take a bit longer to treat. If you are having severe fluctuations in your blood sugar levels, you must consult your doctor. Ignoring it can have serious health repercussions.

Constipation for Long

If the problem of constipation persists for long, you must consult a doctor. It can be due to some other issues too. Ignoring the problem as a normal symptom can be dangerous.

Any Persistent Problem

Most of the symptoms stated above should subside within a week or a fortnight. But, if any problem persists for longer than that, you must consult a doctor and try to find the real reason behind the problem. Intermittent fasting doesn't have any long-term side effect of this nature.

The Ugly

Developing Eating Disorders

This is a problem that some people can face. The chances are rare, but every person has a unique system, and some may react adversely to the changes. If you have had any eating disorders in the past, then you should avoid following intermittent fasting without consulting your doctor.

Persistent Problems Related to Health

If there is any health issue that you are facing despite taking all the care, then you should stop intermittent fasting and observe if the symptoms subside. If that happens, you should stop following intermittent fasting and ask for your doctor's advice.

Chapter 13: Myths and Misconceptions About Intermittent Fasting

Myths and misconceptions have an uncanny way of entering into the common belief. They have no basis, but they are repeated so many times that people start believing in them as truth. Every concept has been marred by these beliefs. Intermittent fasting is a proven way to reap a number of health benefits. You will be eating no pills that may cause side effects. You will not be subjecting yourself to any undue pressure that may cause any harm. Intermittent fasting is a simple way of improving your lifestyle and eating habits.

Given below are some common misconceptions about intermittent fasting that have no scientific basis.

Breakfast Is the Most Important Meal of the Day—Skipping It Will Make You Fat

This a statement every child grows up listening from parents, and it gets imbibed in the head as truth. Breakfast is the meal of the day which you take after breaking your nightly fast. There is nothing to prove that it needs to be early in the morning.

It is a fact that the first meal of the day should be heavy and balanced as it would help you in kickstarting your day. However, it can be taken at any time you like and having it early in the morning is not necessary.

As far as having a balanced and heavy breakfast is concerned, it is important. The reason is that you will be entering into the active part of the day with this meal. If you have a heavy and balanced breakfast, you will be able to push your cravings to have another meal as far as possible. If your breakfast is light, you may start feeling hungry very soon.

Pushing your breakfast to later part of the day will not have anything to do with your being fat. In fact, extending your fasting period will give you weight loss benefits.

You Must Eat Frequently to Keep Your Metabolism Running

This is a myth that has only benefitted the food manufacturing companies. Frequent meals have nothing to do with metabolism. The origin of this concept lies in the fact that your body uses up some energy in processing food. So, if you keep eating frequently, your metabolism will keep working and would burn more energy.

However, it doesn't take into account the fact that you will be consuming more energy than you will burn if you keep having meals at frequent intervals. The energy needed to metabolize the food is only 10–12% of the energy consumed. You will be piling up yourself by eating frequently.

Studies have clearly shown that people who follow intermittent fasting have up to 14% higher metabolism rate than those who don't.

Small Meals at Frequent Intervals Are Important for Losing Weight

This is also a continuation of the earlier myth and has no scientific basis. In fact, science has proven that the higher the number of meals, the greater would be fat storage would be as your insulin would keep storing the excess energy as fat. If you keep having meals at frequent intervals, your fat burning hormones will never be able to work at all.

Brain Will Stop Functioning Without Glucose

It is a fact that brain functions on glucose. However, it is a half baked truth that if you stop consuming carbs, your body would not have any other way to produce glucose. Your body has passed through thousands of years of evolutionary process. It makes no sense to believe that if one type of fuel source is cut off, it wouldn't be able to produce energy through other means.

Your body also has glycogen stores that can be used as energy. Then your body starts using ketones for energy, and your brain would never face a lack of energy to run itself. The brain is the most important organ of the body. It also controls all other functions in the body. It is also one organ that is made of pure fat. Your body serves your brain with complete devotion, and it would always supply it with the required energy either you consume carbs or not.

Our ancestors didn't have access to carbs. They solely relied on fat and protein. Their brains should have stopped functioning thousands of years ago if that was the case.

This is pure myth. Starvation mode is a survival mechanism of your body. Your body enters that starvation mode when it senses a complete energy supply cut off for very long. It takes 72–96 hours for the starvation mode to kick in. In this stage, your body lowers the metabolic rate and starts running only the crucial functions so that it can survive for the longest on the current energy reserves. The body of a healthy adult can run for months in starvation mode. For an obese person, this time can be even longer as the energy reserves are high.

However, the theory that starvation mode would kick in after short fasts have no scientific and reasonable basis. If that would have been the case, our ancestors wouldn't have survived for this long. They needed to be quicker and sharper after short fasting intervals as they needed to put more effort into catching the prey. Short fasts making them slow neither has evolutionary backing nor does it qualify on reason.

Studies have shown that after short fasts, your hGH levels can shoot up several times. In men, the hGH levels can rise up to 2000%, and in women, they can rise up to 1400%. The metabolic rate also goes up by 14%. The adrenaline production in your body also increases considerably. All these things show that you would be more alert, conscious, and active after short fasts.

You Will Lose Muscle Mass if You Follow Intermittent Fasting

People believe that fasting would start cannibalization of the muscles as soon as your blood glucose levels go down. This is a fear that also has no basis. It is a fact that your body first consumes the glucose and then it starts to look for a similar source like protein. However, it doesn't mean that it will eat up all the muscles. Muscles are important for survival your body knows better. Once your glucose supply ends, your body starts looking for alternative energy sources. Some damaged muscles can be used up but that is a part of the cleaning process. However, muscles cannot provide the kind of energy your body needs. It soon starts using fat stores for producing energy which is a steady and better source.

Some loss of muscles would take place with any kind of calorie restrictive regimen. However, the risk of this happening with intermittent fasting is a lot less as it forces and trains your body to burn fat. In fact, with the help of exercise, you can build more muscles than you lose. It is the main reasons that bodybuilders around the globe use intermittent fasting as a bulking routine.

Intermittent Fasting Will Lead to Binge Eating

This a problem that people face more with other diets and calorie restrictive routines than they with intermittent fasting.

Intermittent fasting puts no specific restriction on the number of calories you can eat or even the type of things you can eat. Therefore, the chances of temptation building and cravings are low. You always have the option to eat almost anything in your feasting window as long as you remain in a limit.

This isn't the case with people on diets and calorie restrictive routines as they severely limit the number of calories that can be consumed or the things you can eat. This leads to building up of temptation. You are always thinking about certain food items that you can't eat. As soon as they get a chance, they start eating in an uncontrollable manner and it leads to binge eating. It is one of the reasons people on diets gain more weight that they had lost when they went on diet.

Conclusion

Thanks for making it through to the end of this book. Let's hope it was informative and able to provide you with all of the tools you need to achieve your goals whatever they may be.

This book has been a very sincere effort in providing comprehensive information about the concept of Intermittent Fasting.

It is a concept that has garnered a lot of attention due to its amazing health benefits. However, there is still a lot of confusion about the subject in public.

People try to follow this amazing routine but are unable to get the benefits due to their inability to understand the fine things in the concept.

This book has tried to explain all the aspects of intermittent fasting so that you can reap the maximum benefits out of it.

I hope that you will be able to benefit from this book and lead a healthy and fulfilling life.

Finally, if you found this book useful in any way, a review on Amazon is always appreciated!

9 781798 674161